FITNESS OVER 50 FOR WOMEN

It's Never Too Late To Feel Younger and Improve Your Health. Achieve These Goals With Simple Exercises Illustrated With Explanatory Figures Will Be Much Easier

by Amanda Key

Disclaimer

All erudition supplied in this book is specified for educational and academic purpose only. The author is not in any way in charge for any outcomes that emerge from utilizing this book. Constructive efforts have been made to render information that is both precise and effective, however the author is not to be held answerable for the accuracy or use/misuse of this information.

Table of Contents

Introduction

Life goes too fast. The older you get, the more you will realize how important it is to make the most of each day. So how would you like to slow down the aging process? While we can't go back in time, we can turn the years back on our body with exercise.

Research has shown that exercise can slow the physiological aging clock. That's right, training can keep you young.

And while cardiovascular exercises such as walking, jogging or cycling are important for heart and lung efficiency, it is strength training that provides the benefits that keep your body younger, stronger and more functional as every year passes. If you want to be live and independent for many years, this muscle strengthening workout will help you achieve just that.

Chapter 1: Benefits of weight training

Why should you start lifting weights? Aspect aside, there are many physical, mental, and emotional health benefits associated with weight lifting. In addition to improving your strength, an expected benefit that most people think of when it comes to weight training, there are numerous other physical benefits, such as increased bone density, metabolic rate, cognitive ability, coordination and stability, cardiovascular capacity, energy and cellular function, as well as reducing stress. All of these benefits help you feel strong both physically and mentally and help you the way you see each day. Below are the details and science that support each of these impressive benefits.

1.   More strength. By lifting weights, you will develop the muscle strength needed to lift heavier objects inside and outside the gym. Think about how much easier tasks like carrying groceries and picking up your kids and pets with strong muscles would be! Having stronger muscles will also help maintain an upright posture and support the bone structure.

2.   Increased bone density. Speaking of bones, many women are at risk of developing osteopenia or osteoporosis, the weakening of the bones with age. Weight lifting can help maintain strong bones as you age by increasing bone density. Working the muscles attached to the bones forces your body to lay down more bone-making materials, which strengthens your bones and increases their density. These are two great advantages in one!

3.   Increased metabolic rate. Strength training will also result in more overall muscle mass, and the more muscle you have, the more calories you burn at rest. This is because muscle tissue burns more calories. This means that you will burn extra calories even when you are not exercising simply because you have more muscle mass.

4.   Increased cognitive ability. Basically, strength training makes you smarter. Your brain has to function differently during strength training. It needs to remember movement patterns, know where your limbs are in relation to your body, and pay attention to the stimuli around you. This is a lot of work for your brain, especially if you are new to weight

training. Therefore, it is a great way to train the brain. In addition to making you smarter, weightlifting also helps improve your mood and increases your self-esteem by releasing happiness hormones (endorphins) into your bloodstream.

5.   Greater coordination and stability. Lifting weights and coordinating movements helps you gain better stability, coordination, and proprioceptive feedback (the way your brain recognizes where your body and limbs are during movements). This is useful for avoiding awkward moments or falling.

6.   Increased cardiovascular capacity. Weight training may not sound like cardio, but it's when you train at an intensity that your heart rate increases. It is rhythmic in nature and repeat the movements of the exercises several times. In addition, the heart rate remains increased when passing exercises, i.e. performing back-to-back movements with little or no rest between them. This makes weight lifting a form of cardio (and a lot less boring than using cardio equipment!).

7.   More energy. Weight lifting releases hormones in your body that signal your brain to wake up. These happy

endorphins give you a natural energy boost. That's why many people like to lift weights in the morning or during their lunch breaks to get some energy before starting the day or getting back to work.

8. Better cellular functions. Weight lifting increases blood lactate concentrations, hemoglobin levels and the capillary / fiber ratio in cells. These increases allow cells to function more efficiently by causing blood to flow more fluidly throughout the body. With increased blood flow efficiency, the supply of oxygen and nutrients to the muscles increases and creates optimal cellular performance.

9. Stress reduction. Weightlifting helps you relieve stress by giving your brain and body a way to externalize repressed emotions. The hormones released when you exercise help your body counteract the hormone cortisol that causes stress. Plus, with weight lifting, you build confidence and self-esteem, which also reduce stress. So not only can you shed some weight to feel better and relieve tension, but you also get a healthy dose of stress relieving hormones to relax your brain and improve your confidence after training.

Identify your goals

Now that you know some of the great benefits of training, it's time for you to decide on a goal. Setting a goal drives personal motivation and satisfaction. First, you must start by choosing a goal that is deeply rooted in your "WHY". Your why is something that is very important to you. It is not something superficial or superficial. Rather, your WHY is something that has a personal emotional trigger associated with it - a deep internal motivation that is unique to you. If your goal does not have a WHY associated with it, you will be less likely to succeed.

Also, you need to want to achieve that goal for yourself, not because someone else gave you a goal.

The next step is to make sure your goal is SMART, which means it's specific, measurable, attainable, realistic, and time sensitive. For example, a SMART goal might be "I want to lose 10 pounds in 2 months so that I can participate in more activities during my next family vacation. I'll achieve this by lifting weights 3 times a week." Losing 10 pounds in 2 months is a lot. specific, measurable and achievable within the established time frame. It is also realistic that this person can lift weights 3 times a week. Now, to take the SMART goal one step further, the WHY associated with it could be."

LIVE LONG AND STRONG

We are told that we need to strengthen our bodies, but it is not always clear why muscle strength is so important. In this chapter I will analyze the reasons why we need to maintain, and in many cases rebuild, our muscle mass.

Maybe you thought those people who go to the gym were only there for the sake of vanity. It couldn't be further from the truth. There are numerous reasons why strength training is critical to our health, and it's time we better understand why.

TIME, YOUR BODY AND THE SECRET WEAPON

Physically inactive people will begin to lose a small percentage of muscle every decade after age 30, which contributes to general weakness and lower quality of life. This is a natural process known as sarcopenia. Many people believe that activities like walking, cycling, or swimming will be enough to keep muscles strong. But is not so. While these activities are certainly helpful, they are not enough to keep muscle mass intact.

Adding resistance training will maintain your strength, improve your appearance, balance and posture, and allow you to continue doing the activities you enjoy.

We need to place a new demand on our muscles so that they get the signal you demand the most from them. I love the phrase "Change doesn't happen in your comfort zone," and this is as true for muscle building as it is for our personal growth.

After training with increased resistance, your body repairs and replaces damaged muscle fibers; but the great thing is that this muscle rebuilds itself stronger than before to meet the new needs. Change does not happen overnight, but it will happen. As I often tell my clients, your body can't help but get stronger if you keep making these demands on it safely and consistently.

Muscle knows no age, but the sooner you start, the better the quality of life you will have at 40, 50, 60 and beyond!

THE MUSCLE CONNECTION, HORMONE AND METABOLISM

Strength training triggers the production of the hormones that control our metabolism and help us develop muscles. We are learning that our musculoskeletal system acts as a kind of endocrine organ that plays a key role in metabolism.

In recent years, the hormones insulin and cortisol have become part of the body composition conversation. We began to realize that getting lean isn't as simple as "calories in versus calories out". When it comes to changing the fat-to-muscle ratio, both calories and hormones matter, particularly as we age. Even though we need to be in a calorie deficit (absorbing fewer calories than we're burning) for your stored energy to be used as fuel, managing cravings when we're trying to cut calories has more to do with hormones.

The fact that strength training can lower insulin levels means that levels can normalize while cortisol is kept in check. Since there appears to be a connection between cortisol and estrogen dominance (which can worsen for many women as we approach menopause), it is important to keep both insulin and cortisol in normal ranges. When cortisol is elevated for long periods of time, it can cause negative health problems, including increased abdominal fat.

Older people tend to be more insulin resistant, but the reasons for this are controversial. Is it an inevitable part of aging or the result of lifestyle choices? Personally, I'd wager that insulin resistance has more to do with lifestyle choices and is responsible for the increased risk of type 2 diabetes, as well as heart attacks, strokes and cancer.

The bottom line is that strength training is the most powerful tool for building muscle and losing fat. There are no alternatives and no shortcuts. By putting our body back together in this way, we will be able to better manage our hormone levels and keep that complicated endocrine system in great order as we age. Furthermore, there is the fundamental fact that muscle burns more calories than fat. This means that the more muscle tissue you have, the more calories your body burns, even at rest.

BONE DENSITY

Most people know that strength training, whether with bodyweight, dumbbells, barbells, kettlebells, or resistance bands, can build muscle and strength. But did you know that by strengthening our muscles we also strengthen our bones, which in turn helps to minimize osteoporosis? Osteoporosis is the loss of calcium and other minerals from a person's bones, which makes the bones susceptible to fracture.

A sedentary lifestyle is the main contributing factor to bone loss as we age. Bone loss is estimated at a rate of about one percent per year after age 40 or so, if we don't intentionally work against it. The more significant the loss of bone density, the more susceptible we are to fracturing a bone, even while performing a simple task.

The great news is that strength training can seriously slow bone loss, and as some studies have shown, it can even rebuild bone. When I first consult with a new client who has been diagnosed with osteopenia or osteoporosis, I am always happy to learn that their doctor has recommended strength training, rather than putting them on medication or just recommending a calcium supplement.

A "load exercise" is a form of exercise that will help compensate for osteoporosis. The loading activity places stress on the bones by creating a traction action, which in turn can stimulate the growth of bone cells. The best way to create this jerk action is through strength training, although you will get some benefits with aerobic activities such as walking, hiking, jogging, playing racquet sports, and even dancing. However, if you have a serious concern about bone loss, strength training has the greatest regenerative effect by targeting your bones in a targeted way.

One of the most moving parts of my job is seeing my clients gain the wonderful sense of confidence that comes from acquiring a stronger, more stable body. This confidence appears to propel them into new activities and serves to satisfy the social and emotional aspects of their life as well as their physical fitness.

STRENGTH, BALANCE AND MOBILITY

Strength, together with balance, affects our ability to move in a functional way; therefore, if our mobility is limited, due to decreased balance and strength, we will be at risk for the general deterioration of our structural bodies, as well as the emotional components that are likely to accompany the loss of function.

If we allow our muscles to atrophy to the point of noticeable muscle loss and weakness, then balance and mobility will suffer.

Good balance requires coordination of different parts of the body, including muscles, bones and joints. There are also other problems that can affect balance, such as vision or inner ear problems, but if we maintain our strength and range of motion, we will be less prone to losing balance in the first place and better able. to recover if we do. Balance with advancing age is essential. A major cause of injury to older people is falls.

The combination of strength, balance and mobility equals stability and stability equals a strong and sturdy body. Strengthening movements with free weights require stability so that the stabilizing muscles have to step in to help and, in turn, become stronger, along with the targeted muscle group. For example, by doing exercises one leg at a time, you need to keep your balance for even just a second or two, which requires the use of our hip stabilizers. By incorporating hip stabilizers, we not only strengthen the muscles surrounding the hip joints, but help create a more stable body overall.

These days there isn't as much emphasis on flexibility as it once was. Instead, we focus on maintaining our natural range of motion in combination with strength. While it is important to maintain our natural range of motion, stretching beyond that point can do more harm than good. An increase in flexibility without force results in joint instability. So once again we see the importance of keeping our muscles strong.

HEALTH OF THE BRAIN

In recent years, various studies have shown that greater muscle strength is associated with better cognitive function in men and women as they age. Cognition refers to the brain functions related to receiving, storing, processing and using information. These results were published in the European Geriatric Medicine Journal.

Scientists at Florida Atlantic University have found that sarcopenia and obesity (independently, but especially if they occur together) can increase the risk of cognitive function disorders later in life. These results were published in the journal Clinical Interventions in Aging. Meanwhile, a 2012 University of British Columbia study published in the Archives of Internal Medicine compared cardio exercise and strength training in a randomized, controlled trial. Neuroimaging of the brain showed that the areas responsible for memory and executive function were most active after strength training.

This study showed that seniors who did both cardio and strength exercises were generally healthier than those who only did yoga and pilates. But the most significant finding from this study was that those people who did most of the weight training showed significantly fewer brain injuries. The study concluded that weight lifting is beneficial for overall brain health.

It's safe to say that strength training is good for us for so many reasons, including having neuroprotective properties.

Lifting weights not only helps us regain physical strength and increase our metabolism, it also helps us maintain a healthy brain!

It is important to take responsibility for learning about fitness and nutrition, because knowledge really is power. Our bodies are amazing machines and the more we learn about how they work, the more likely we are to take care of them.

Remember that there is no magic pill, potion or product that will do the job for you. In the beginning, there will be some trial and error as you embark on your new lifestyle. When you make a mistake or fall off the fitness bandwagon, forgive yourself. Get up, dust off and keep moving forward.

Chapter 2: NUTRITION

It is impossible to discuss strength training without addressing nutrition. A common saying you'll hear at the gym is "You can't get over a bad diet." If we continue to consume too many nutrient-empty calories in the form of processed sugary "foods" without the right balance of macronutrients, our efforts with strength training will end in frustration. For example, a 150-pound person would have to run for about 45 minutes or lift weights vigorously for about 50 minutes to burn 500 calories. It would be infinitely easier to replace that 500-calorie muffin with an apple, but it's not just about limiting calories for fat loss. Proper nutrition also means creating the necessary environment to build and strengthen our muscles,

Micro and macronutrients

Micronutrients are vitamins and minerals that our body needs to stay healthy. They play an important role in human development and well-being, including the regulation of metabolism, heart rate and bone density. They can be found in fruits, vegetables, nuts, dairy, and organ meats, among other sources.

Macronutrients are proteins, carbohydrates and fats. A good ratio for muscle building is 25% protein, 55% carbohydrates and 20% fat, for both men and women. Some nutritionists recommend a ratio of 40% carbohydrates, 30% protein and 30% fat as a good goal for healthy weight loss. To function optimally, our body needs a good balance of micro and macronutrients.

Protein

Protein (1 gram = 4 calories) is a key nutrient for gaining strength and size, losing fat and controlling hunger.

To gain muscle mass, the recommendation for active adults is to consume between 1.2 and 1.7 grams of protein per kilogram of target body weight per day, or 0.5 to 0.8 grams per pound of target body weight.

Based on a (low) daily calorie intake of 1500 calories, your protein intake should be between 375 and 450 calories, with the highest amount recommended for weight loss. For reference, a chicken leg contains 13.5 grams of protein and about 110 calories.

Carbohydrates

Carbohydrates (1 gram = 4 calories) often get a bad rap, especially when it comes to weight gain. But carbohydrates aren't all bad. They provide fuel for the brain and energy for our muscles. In general, carbohydrates should make up about 40-45% of your daily calorie intake for weight loss and 55-60% for maintenance.

It is important to stick to complex carbohydrates rather than simple carbohydrates. Simple carbohydrates are "foods" with added sugar and refined grains, such as sugary drinks, desserts, and candy, which are high in unnecessary calories.

Examples of complex carbohydrates are:

» Fruit rich in fiber (raspberries, apples, avocados)

» Vegetables (broccoli, acorn squash, peas, Brussels sprouts)

» Nuts (almonds, pine nuts, pistachios)

» Whole grains (bulgur, barley, amaranth, rye)

» Seeds (chia, flax, sesame)

» Legumes (lima beans, lentils, beans)

Fat

Dietary fats (1 gram = 9 calories) provide energy and aid in nutrient absorption, as well as brain and nerve function. Some unsaturated fatty acids are essential nutrients, which means that we need to get these fats from food because our bodies cannot produce them. Fats and oils also add flavor and make you feel full for longer and should make up about 20 percent of your daily calorie intake.

The two types of fat are saturated and unsaturated. Saturated fats are solid at room temperature while unsaturated fats are liquid. Unsaturated fats are considered the healthiest type of dietary fat. Choosing unsaturated rather than saturated fats can help reduce the risk of heart disease and stroke.

Pre-Workout Nutrition Ideas

LIGHT MEALS

Depending on the timing of your workout, you may want to have a small meal an hour before your workout rather than an energy snack. Your small meal should consist of equal parts lean protein and carbohydrates. Examples included:

» Two hard-boiled eggs with whole meal toast and sliced tomatoes

» Whey protein shake isolate with fruit, including ½ banana, berries or apples

» Brown rice or long grain white rice with half chicken breast or steamed salmon and broccoli

» Small bowl of wheat pasta with tomato and ⅓ cup of ragù

» Salad, cucumber, tomatoes, bell pepper, dried cranberries with ½ cup diced chicken

» Whole meal bagel with smoked salmon, thinly sliced onion and a thin layer of cream cheese

» Vegan kale Caesar salad with tempeh bacon

» Chicken breast and baked potato stuffed with asparagus

» Greek salad with half grilled chicken breast

» Mediterranean couscous salad with lemon, feta, olive and chickpea aromatic herb dressing

SNACKS

Eating lightly about half an hour before training will allow you to enter with maximum energy. Combining a complex carbohydrate with a lean protein is the best way to fuel your body.

Examples included:

» A banana with almond butter

» Multigrain crackers with hummus

» Whole meal bread with unsweetened peanut butter

» ½ cup of oatmeal with raisins or berries

» Rice cake with peanut butter and sliced apple

» Bowl of plain Greek yogurt with blueberries and granola

Post-workout nutritional ideas

LIGHT MEALS

In general, we want to eat a combination of protein, fat and carbohydrates before and after our workouts, but our pre-workout should be more carb-dense and our post-workout nutrition should be higher in protein. Examples included:

» Grilled chicken with roasted vegetables

» Two egg omelette with roasted vegetables and whole meal toast

» 6 ounces of beef tenderloin with brown rice and broccoli

»Salmon with quinoa and green beans

» Shrimps, egg pasta and green salad dressed with oil and vinegar

» Pork fillet with roasted vegetables and sweet potatoes

» Avocado and tomato on whole meal or sourdough toast with Havarti cheese

» Burrito with beans, brown rice, guacamole and salsa

» Tofu with mushrooms and broccoli

» Chicken salad with mixed vegetables, tomatoes, peppers, onions and spinach dressed with lemon and olive oil

SNACKS

For those times when you just need to recharge after a workout but aren't ready for a full meal:

» Goat cheese, rice crackers and olives

» Ricotta and fruit

» Pita and hummus

» Protein smoothie with Greek yogurt and berries

» Handful of almonds or walnuts with goji berries

Hydration

Drinking fluids is critical to staying healthy for every system in your body. The fluids carry nutrients to the cells, eliminate bacteria from the bladder and prevent constipation.

In general, you should drink 16 to 32 ounces of fluid every 60 minutes while exercising. For exercises that last less than an hour, drink only water. However, if it's excessively hot or humid, a sports drink can be a healthy option. For exercise lasting over an hour, drink water, a high-quality sports drink, or both for optimal hydration.

Supplements

First of all, do your best to get the nutrients from your foods. However, you may want to supplement your diet if you suspect you are not getting enough with the food you eat.

B12

Your body uses vitamin B12 to fight germs and to produce energy. You need more B12 as you get older. Help your body make red blood cells, which are responsible for supplying oxygen to the muscles.

Calcium and Magnesium

Together, magnesium and calcium are essential for bone health. Without magnesium, calcium can become toxic to the kidneys, arteries and cartilage, instead of depositing in the bones where it is needed most.

Vitamin D

This vitamin helps you absorb calcium and can help prevent osteoporosis. It also helps the function of muscles, nerves and the immune system. Most people get some vitamin D from sunlight, but our bodies are less able to convert the sun's rays into vitamin D as we age.

Fish oil

The fatty acids contained in fish oil have several benefits for building muscle, such as reducing muscle pain. The American

Heart Association recommends that people with coronary artery disease take omega-3 fatty acids (the kind found in fish) to prevent heart attacks.

Protein powder

If you feel you are having trouble eating enough protein, you may want to invest in a good protein powder. The various protein powders on the market are one way to make sure you are getting enough protein to effectively build muscle. There are also some vegan options on the market. Add a scoop to a smoothie and you'll be good to go!

Chapter 3: YOUR EQUIPMENT AND YOUR GYM

This book will provide you with both home workouts that you can do with a few tools, and workouts you can do in the gym, if that's your preference. If there are days when you can't go to the gym or you prefer to exercise at home, it is helpful to have two or three varieties of dumbbell weights and strengths and / or resistance bands.

Some people start strength training by doing bodyweight exercises at home and then progress over time to using weights and / or resistance bands. Bodyweight exercises are a great place to start, but remember that your body won't get stronger if you don't progressively add resistance.

Resistance bands

These exercise bands are useful tools to take your workout with you while traveling. My clients travel a lot and love to take their bands with them on their adventures to maintain their strength during their absence. Band exercises are surprisingly effective and inexpensive. Anything you can do with dumbbells, you can do with these bands.

Dumbbells

If you work out at home, refer to Chapter 5 for weight tips. You may soon find that you've headed back to the sporting goods store looking for heavier dumbbells as your body gets stronger. Basically, you will use lighter weights for your smaller muscles (like arms and shoulders) and heavier weights for your bigger muscles (like chest, back and legs).

Shoes

For both home and gym, make sure you have a good pair of sneakers. I am a fan of the lighter sports shoes rather than the chunky trainers with very thick soles that you can find on the market. However, if you have foot problems and have been specifically advised by your doctor, be sure to follow their footwear advice. If you are a runner and have specific running shoes, feel free to wear them while lifting weights.

Bottle of water

I suggest you keep a refillable water bottle with you while exercising and throughout the day. This way you can keep track of your hydration and avoid potential dehydration or even heat exhaustion.

Gloves

You may also want to invest in a pair of heavy duty weight lifting gloves to keep your palms callus free.

REST AND RECOVERY

You may hear about the importance of exercise and the negative effects of inactivity, but it's not that common to hear why you also need to give your body time to rest. Rest is just as important as muscle building training.

Rest

Getting enough rest between workouts allows your muscles to rebuild and regenerate before the next session. The recommended amount of rest time between strength sessions targeting the same muscle groups is 48 hours. But "rest" doesn't mean we don't move at all. On your days off, go for a nice walk, take a Zumba class, or do some restorative yoga.

To sleep

REM (Rapid Eye Movement) sleep is critical for strength training recovery, as it is during this time that human protein synthesis and growth hormones are released, enabling muscle repair and recovery.

With too little sleep, the body is more likely to produce the stress hormone cortisol. I won't go into the science of all of this, but I know that studies have shown that there is a definite connection between lack of sleep and increased cortisol levels, which can contribute to atrophy in both muscle and bone, as well as weight. I earn.

How to assess the need for recovery

After a good strength training, expect to feel some muscle pain the next day or even two days later. This is called delayed onset muscle pain (DOMS). Rest assured that you will not always feel muscle soreness; but in the beginning, when you push harder, or when you change programs, you will probably feel some muscle pain. This is all normal and perfectly safe.

However, if you feel overly fatigued after a workout, you may have pushed too hard. If that happens, go a little easier next time. Rest, proper nutrition, adequate sleep and continue.

GET PUMPED: GOAL WORKSHEET

I often tell my clients that if they want to be successful in maintaining their motivation in strength training, it is imperative to find their "why". I explain the difference between inspiration and motivation by saying that inspiration comes from without, while motivation comes from within.

Consider asking yourself one of the following if you're looking for your motivation:

» How do I want to interact with my children / grandchildren? Do I want to enjoy the ski slopes or the ocean with them rather than always being on the sidelines as a spectator?

» How do I see my future travels? Am I willing to settle for not being able to climb the hill to see the view, climb around the ruins, or keep up with the tour?

» Am I willing to allow weakened joints to exclude me from my favorite hikes and sports?

» I have heard that strength training will help me with my depression / anxiety / mood. Am I willing to try everything I can to naturally elevate my mood?

» I've heard that strength training helps with cognitive health. Am I willing to do whatever I can to keep a healthy brain?

» I want to maintain an active and fun sex life, but am I willing to risk losing it by not maintaining my strength and vital energy?

Chapter 4: When and how often to train

When and how often to train depends on your goals and lifestyle. The important thing is to decide on a routine and stick to it. Check your schedule and realistically determine how many days per week you can commit to training. Decide if morning, afternoon or evening is best for you based on your schedule and energy levels throughout the day. You may also decide that changing the time of day works best for you.

It will not affect the results of your program, as long as you are consistent in training for the number of days you commit. Two days of training a week is the minimum amount you will need to commit to to see changes in your body. At least 3 days is optimal, but some people can endure 4 or 5 days depending on their training style and goals. You may want to consider starting with fewer days and adding more as you build your training program. Being aggressive and starting with too many days can lead to unrealistic expectations and damage your motivation.

You should plan for your workouts to last from 30 to 90 minutes, including warm-up and recovery time. Your goals will determine the length of your weight lifting program. If your goal is to burn fat or lose weight, you should create circuits of 3 or 4 exercises to be performed one after the other for a set. This type of training will include fewer rest breaks and take less time. If you are looking to gain muscle mass, your training will focus on one exercise at a time or supersets with maximum rest and recovery times. This type of training will take longer and may include more exercises to strain a particular muscle group. Another factor that will affect your training time is the number of days you commit to training. If, for example, you train 4 or 5 times a week, so intervals of 30-45 minutes would be a good amount of time to help prevent overtraining. (Overtraining occurs when you train too much and don't get the proper amount of recovery time.) If you're only able to train 2 or 3 times a week, then 60-90 minutes would be ideal for maximizing results, as they are engaging for fewer days.

BEST HEATING PRACTICES

Warming up is an important part of the weight lifting process. It is necessary to ensure that the muscles have adequate blood flow and that the joints are sufficiently lubricated and mobile before loading them with additional weight. This will make your weight lifting sessions more effective and also prevent injuries from occurring. Here are three best practices for getting the most out of your warm-up.

• Warm up the muscles you will be working on. What you include in your warm-up should be based on what you intend to do as a workout that day. For example, if you are working with the upper body, you should include movements that use the arms, such as jumping jacks, bear strips, or boards. If you are working on the lower body, you will include movements like lunges, squats, toe toes, and butt kickers. In the next few exercise chapters, you'll see some suggested warm-up movements that you can use to prepare those specific muscles to work.

• Start increasing your heart rate. Your warm-up should take 5 to 10 minutes. Eventually, you want to feel like you are sweating slightly. You should also have an elevated heart rate at this point, around 115 to 125 beats per minute (bpm). Using cardio equipment, such as jogging or walking up an incline on the treadmill, can definitely help your warm-up. However, you still want to include some specific movements to target the muscle groups you intend to work that day.

•   Use dynamic movements. You want your warm-up to be dynamic. This means you want it to mimic the exercises you plan on doing later in your workout - it should serve as a preparation for movement. For example, standing and reaching towards the toes to stretch the hamstrings is great but not dynamic. A better way to stretch the hamstrings before lifting would be to perform straight leg kicks. The more dynamic a movement is, the more closely related it is to the actions that the leg muscles will need to perform to effectively lift.

THE CRITICAL RELOAD

Post-workout recovery time is just as important as pre-workout warm-up. Just as you need to prepare your muscles and joints for movement, you also need to signal them that they can relax and move blood to other parts of the body. Choose your recovery time based on what you did for a workout. For example, if you've been running your upper body, it may be helpful to passively stretch your back and arms for a few seconds to relieve some of the tension you've built up in them. Passive stretches are great to include in your cooldown. You can hold each stretch for 30-45 seconds. You can also use cardio equipment or take a short walk or very light jog to cool down.

You don't want to skip your cooldown. Even if you are very tired, it is essential to cool your body. (Walking to the car or taking a shower doesn't count.) If you don't, your muscles may feel severe cramps after exercising. Your muscles will also remain in a shortened state, which will negatively impact your joint mobility and posture.

DAYS OF REST AND RECOVERY

Rest and recovery are important to take into account to maximize results. If you don't rest and recover, you risk overtraining. Symptoms of overtraining include getting sick, feeling sore, aches, decreased performance, mood swings, excessive fatigue, insomnia, increased perceived exertion during exercise, and injury.

It is best to have at least 2 days off per week. When you work out with weights, you break down muscle tissue. Therefore, muscles need at least a day to rebuild stronger muscle fibers than before - this process can sometimes take up to 3 days. You will need to be aware of which muscle groups you are working out each day and give each muscle group at least 1 or 2 days to recover. As you progress on your weightlifting journey, you will become more in tune with your body. When this happens, you will be able to gauge how much rest and recovery time you need for each muscle group.

Be aware that you will experience some muscle pain after the first few days of weight lifting. This is called DOMS (delayed onset muscle soreness). It is the period of 24 to 48 hours after weight lifting when the muscles are rebuilding the muscle fibers. The goal is not to be sore after each workout. Eventually, you will find a balance where you feel worked but not overworked after weight lifting. This also comes from being more in tune with your body as you progress.

Weightlifting has many other benefits besides aesthetics. While aesthetics may be the reason you start out or what you feel most about, the other benefits outlined at the beginning of this chapter can bring much more into your life. For this reason, you find that you want to make weight lifting a part of your lifestyle. The key to accomplishing this is to find the other motivating factors that keep you connected to a WHY that goes deeper than appearance. Here are some tips on how to find out those extra motivational factors that will help you maintain a lifting life.

Tip No. 1: do not lift for aesthetic reasons. Looking good is a great way to motivate yourself when you start out, but what happens as you get older? As your body begins to change with age, you may not look the same as before. If you do, great! But your ideal aesthetic is likely to be unmanageable in the long run. Focus on mastering a particular movement that you couldn't do before or on lifting a specific amount of weight. These types of imperative goals are more motivating to get you lifted for life than aesthetics alone.

Tip No. 2: listen to your body. Weight lifting is great, but it puts a strain on your body, so you need to be smart and listen to your body. Make movements that make your body feel good. Also, rest when your body says it needs it.

Tip No. 3: take time to recover. As mentioned above, taking care of your body is very important and there are several things you can do. Spend time each day on stretching and foam rolling, or learn other methods of myofascial release (SMR) for yourself. SMR is the process of removing knots, or trigger points, in the fascia of muscles using various massage techniques and tools. Massages are also helpful in helping your muscles recover and making sure you get enough sleep and water is important.

Tip No. 4: get a personal trainer. A personal trainer can help you keep your routine fresh and not boring. They can also schedule workouts to help you prevent injuries and get proper rest between workouts. Personal trainers are worth the money. There is no price too high to invest in your health.

Tip No. 5: turn it on. Mixing up your routine keeps you from getting bored. As you gain confidence in weight training, try adding different modes and equipment, such as kettlebells, TRX straps (total body resistance exercise), a ViPR (short for "vitality, performance and reconditioning"), resistance, machines, and cables, into your workout routine. Learning to master the movements with new training stimuli will test your brain and body.

Tip No. 6: keep moving. Get inspired to do something every day. Make weight lifting a part of your lifestyle, not a chore. A little movement every day helps you keep what you have, so move it or lose it!

Chapter 5: Why bodyweight training?

The word "workout" most likely conjures up images of a sweaty gym with people huddled on machines and dumbbells moving back and forth. There is no doubt that weight training is effective. I mean, I'm a heavy weightlifter too! However, thinking that it is the only useful form of training is a mistake.

Weightlifting has its positives, but one of the biggest negatives to do with it is the prevalence of injuries. To progress, you need to keep increasing the weight you lift. Eventually there comes a point where you will be close to your maximum strength limit and with the intention of completing your set of exercises you will end up injuring yourself as your body will simply fail.

Injuries sustained from weight lifting can be life-threatening, especially if they involve the joints or back. Injuries aside, it's no secret that these types of exercises place a huge load on your joints ("Most Common Weightlifting Injuries and 5 Tips to Avoid Them", 2019). You will also need tons of equipment to train properly.

The advantages of bodyweight training

This is where bodyweight training is far superior to weight lifting. All you need is your body. You don't need any equipment or accessories. The reason most people find bodyweight training ineffective is that they perform the exercises incorrectly.

For example, one of the most common bodyweight exercises is the pushup. It's pretty simple. Lie on your stomach and push yourself off the ground. You'd be surprised how many people fail to perform this exercise correctly and end up suffering injuries to their shoulders and wrists.

You can be injured from any movement performed incorrectly. The form is what determines the likelihood of injury, not the type of exercise. The sticking point is that the injuries you can potentially sustain when training with just your own body weight will be far less severe than the injuries you sustain while lifting weights. This is because your body is not being pushed too far beyond its limit.

Recovery and energy levels after a workout are on average higher with these types of exercises. There is no need to buy medicine balls or sign up for yoga classes to preserve flexibility unless you want to. Your body will work within safe limits while pushing itself to grow stronger at the same time. Let's take a closer look at some of the benefits of bodyweight training.

You don't need a gym or accessories

This is self-explanatory. You don't need special equipment for a pushup. Some exercises need accessories, but even these are so easy to obtain that it's ridiculous to think of them as accessories. For example, you need a bar of some kind to perform a pullup. This can be a particular accessory you buy, or it can be a monkey bar you find at a playground or at the beach.

It can be a wooden or metal beam in your home or garage. It can be a tree branch. What I mean is that you won't have to spend too much time figuring out how to do the exercise, but I still recommend buying a real pull-up bar for your home.

Excellent weight / power ratio

Here's how progress in weightlifting happens. You lift a certain amount of weight today and tomorrow (or a set time limit later), you lift the weight that is one degree higher than it. The idea is that your muscles are continually tested and need to grow to make progress.

This works for the most part, but the problem is your body isn't a machine. There are days when it's not at its best. There are days when he needs ample rest. Forcing an arbitrary weight number externally will cause injury. Training in this way also assumes that everyone's body responds equally to training routines.

This is simply not true as everyone's body is different. By training with your body weight, you allow your body to adapt and modulate how much energy it can devote to that particular exercise without overloading itself. This prevents many injuries that are common when lifting weights.

Greater flexibility and balance

Thanks to your body having more room to work (in terms of being able to better adapt to the weight it needs to push), you develop more agility and flexibility. Communication between the different parts of the body improves and you will find that you will use your muscles much more efficiently.

For example, once you start doing push-ups, you will notice that your core becomes stronger, even if you are not exercising it directly. This will impact the way you walk and you will find yourself standing straighter because your core now supports you more actively.

Weight training involves many isolation exercises. You can train your biceps to look as beautiful and sturdy as they can be, but when you lift something off the floor, you're using your legs, glutes, back, shoulder, core, and biceps. If these muscles aren't used to talking to each other, the amount of weight you can lift in real life won't be equivalent to the weight you lift in the gym.

Bodyweight training simply avoids all of these problems by never having to isolate anything in the first place. Your sense of balance and flexibility will remain what it was before starting the workout and will also increase.

Clear goals

As your body will be able to adapt much better to your training methods, you will be able to better set and achieve your training goals. A common occurrence in weight training regimes is stalling. This refers to when the trainee cannot lift beyond a certain amount of weight after a while.

Stalling occurs due to fatigue building up over time and the body reaches a level beyond which it cannot move forward without significant rest. Most trainees have no idea how to run the stalls and it takes some experience to get through them. There is no risk of stalling with bodyweight training as you are always within the limits of your body.

In fact, it sets the speed of progress and the tone of your workout. Therefore, your goals are much clearer and you never have any doubts about which level to aim for.

Variations

Our bodies are incredibly versatile and can adapt to many situations. Once you start exercising, you will realize that your body will adapt and get used to that movement. As a result, progress occurs in shorter bursts and it will take you longer to see the same level of gains you experienced previously.

When this happens with weight training, you will need to understand different exercises to perform, which means learning new movements. With bodyweight training, adjustments are much easier to make. Sticking to the pushup, if you find that your body is adjusting, lift one of your legs off the floor the next time you do it.

Even better, place your legs on an elevation and push up from a decline. You can do the Rocky Balboa pushup where you bend over with one arm, explode up and down with the other and repeat the action. You can bring your arms closer to your body or push harder. Lift both legs off the ground, etc. Etc. There is almost no end to the number of variations you can field when training this way. All this allows you to continue surprising your body and you will make more steady and consistent progress.

Tailored

Bodyweight training is an extremely flexible and versatile training method. Through such routines, you will be able to work towards multiple goals simultaneously as it helps develop your strength, stamina and agility (Why bodyweight training, 2019). Also, if you are looking to take on a new sport, bodyweight training has a number of benefits for you as it will provide a solid foundation for any other form of activity.

Chapter 6: The most common training mistakes and how to avoid them

One of the reasons why most exercise regimens fail is because people make highly avoidable mistakes. Many of these apply equally to bodyweight training routines. With that in mind, let's take a look at some of the mistakes you should avoid.

Training beyond capacity

This mistake is almost impossible to make when training with body weight, but it still occurs. The most common way is when the trainee decides to get creative with his or her workout and shoves a dumbbell or plate of additional weights onto the exercise and suddenly the body is pushed beyond its capabilities. Practice until failure

Unlike the previous mistake, this is absolutely possible when you only train with your own body weight. This occurs mainly due to the stereotype surrounding hard training. Common motivational sayings like "go hard or go home" and so on make people think that unless they throw up their guts, they haven't really worked out.

The truth is that the ideal strength level you want to achieve is about 90% of your maximum capacity. This means that you should stop performing the exercise when you feel that you will be fighting within a couple of extra reps. Of course, this is a feeling-based metric that will be difficult to understand at first. However, over time you will get to know your body better and avoid this mistake.

Lack of a plan

How many times have you seen people dress in their fancy workout clothes once they hit the gym, and all they do is randomly train on various things before packing to go home at the slightest hint of sweat? The thing is, you need to plan your gym workout long before you decide to go into it.

This means having a clear and precise training plan that lists how many reps or the interval for which you will perform an exercise. Not only does this schedule need to be done for a daily session, but also between sessions. How will you make sure you keep pushing yourself to the ideal limit?

This is where a workout routine helps immensely. It doesn't have to be luxurious, but you do need a basic plan in place. Anything else and you will end up looking clueless.

Too many repetitions

Rep is short for repetition and high repetition exercises are one of the most common mistakes made by beginners. It's not just beginners, even people who have been training unsuccessfully for a while end up making this mistake. The reason this error occurs is that most people don't understand that training methods depend on goals.

To be honest, the weightlifting world is more susceptible to this than bodyweight trainers. What usually happens is that a beginner goes to the gym and sees the carcass in the corner, lifting small weights for a large number of repetitions. The reason the Hulk trains this way is because he already has a high level of strength and these low weight / high rep routines give him good pump.

A beginner will see no benefit from these routines as they have no muscles to pump in the first place. They have to work to build their strength before worrying about what they will look like. When doing bodyweight exercises, you need to focus on pushing your strength forward as much as possible instead of trying to do too many repetitions for one exercise.

Ignore illness or injury

One of the most perverse outcomes that create motivational speeches and quotes is getting sick people to work out instead of staying home and getting better. Trying to train when you're sick is a bit like trying to run with a bad leg. You just won't do it very well.

Even worse, training and exercise put stress on the body, and when you are sick, stress is the last thing you need. So be kind to yourself and let it go for a while. Injury is a difficult thing for most beginners because they cannot distinguish between pain and injury.

Pain is the result of a lack of blood flow through a particular area, while injury is the result of tissue damage. The former always feels uncomfortable but disappears once you perform the same movement that caused it, thus forcing blood to flow through the muscle again. An injury will always be accompanied by severe pain or pain when attempting to perform the movement that caused it. You will also feel weakness in that area when you move it around.

Learning to identify the difference between pain and injury takes time. The key is to minimize the risk of injury before learning the difference.

Inadequate rest

Regardless of the routine you choose to follow, you need an adequate amount of rest. This usually allows for a 24 hour rest period between your workouts. As you become more experienced, you can shorten it as you will get to know your body better. However, in the beginning, it is best to train every other day, especially when you are looking to increase strength.

Rest periods are extremely important because real progress occurs when you rest, not when you exercise. It is during the rest period that your body repairs itself and breaks down existing muscle fibers to build larger and stronger ones. This is where strength is built. So never underestimate your rest periods and always prioritize.

Lack of heating

Have you ever tried to start a car in the middle of winter? Or have you ever tried to accelerate it to full speed right after starting the engine? If your car is brand new, it won't need much of a warm-up period, but the engine is unlikely to reach peak performance immediately. An old machine could die on you if you try to.

Your body is more or less the same. By the way, I'm not saying you'll die from a lack of heat. What I mean is that you need to take the time to get the blood flowing to various parts of your body before pushing it close to the limit. This is common sense, but most people who train don't follow this simple rule.

They jump in and immediately try to lift the weight they should be lifting during that session. This is the easiest way to hurt yourself. You may have gotten away with it when you were younger, but trying to do it at your current age is a terrible idea.

Ignore nutrition

When you exercise, you burn calories. Your body is under stress and needs food (fuel) to recover. Not eating well and eating inadequate amounts of food is one of the most significant mistakes participants make. To be honest, this error usually occurs due to a lack of planning.

Plan your meals in advance so you don't go home to an empty kitchen or refrigerator after training. Grabbing a fast food after training might be okay once or twice, but you don't want to get used to it. Remember that as you get older, you will need to pay more attention to the micronutrients in your food, such as vitamins and minerals.

Junk food is full of processed chemicals that give you a short-term sugar rush but nothing in the way of nutrition. So plan your meals and quantities in advance and make sure you don't go hungry and undo all your progress.

Improper macros

Macros refer to macronutrients. There are three of them, namely proteins, fats and carbohydrates. Protein is needed to build muscle while fat and carbohydrates are fuel for your body. Trying to train and exercise without eating the right amount of carbohydrates and fats is a bit like trying to drive a vehicle without gas.

There is a lot of literature on proper nutrition breakdown and so on, but the best way to make sure you are eating the right amount of nutrients is to follow a balanced diet. This way, you are guaranteed to be getting the right levels of nutrition.

Don't vary your workouts

I mentioned earlier that our bodies are incredibly adaptable and can adapt to any workout or activity level over time. Once they adapt, they consume less energy to do that activity. The result is that your progress rate will slow down. The best way to avoid this is to change routines and keep the body guessed right.

There is a danger of going to the other extreme and varying your workouts too much. I'm not saying you should be doing something different every day, but an excellent way to determine when it's time for a change is to check yourself for boredom. When you feel it happening, switch things up and charge your body again.

Lack of monitoring and measurement

If you've worked out before, have you ever hit the gym with a notepad and pen and keep track of how much and what you lifted? Chances are you've never done this. This is quite normal for all trainees. They assume that adopting a workout routine somehow ensures they will make progress and fail to realize that in order to progress, you need to measure and monitor performance. When you start your training session, you should know exactly what you will do, as well as the duration and amount of time you will do it for. Your training log contains all of this information and you should keep track of everything you do. Think of it as your progress log.

Poor form

Many beginners rush into their workout routine full of energy and excitement and get injured promptly. This is due to the fact that they practice improper form. The form here refers to the technique of the exercise. For example, if you are doing the pushup, you need to make sure your back stays straight and is not bent. This is a simple instruction, but in an attempt to squeeze that extra repetition, some people tend to bend their backs.

With bodyweight exercises, improper form will not result in massive injuries. However, this doesn't mean you should ignore the form. Proper form ensures that you develop strength the right way and hit the right muscles when performing the exercise. Thus, in addition to preventing personal injury, the shape also guarantees a good level of strength and endurance. Isolation is too early

As I said earlier, huge guys in the gym tend to do isolation exercises because they're tied to their goals (Why bodyweight training, 2019). Their goals are very different from yours, and as such, it makes no sense for you to follow their lead. Isolation exercises are best for those who are looking to give their muscles better shape.

They are not really geared towards building overall strength. To be effective, the trainee must have a fair amount of muscle to begin with. At that stage, an isolation routine will help them develop both the form and the other lifts because it will ensure that every muscle in the muscle chain is as strong as possible.

Strength training is what makes the muscles talk to each other and work in tandem. It is useless to strengthen a part of the chain when the chain itself barely exists. So, focus on the basics of strength first and worry about form later. You will look good once you reach a decent strength level, so don't worry about that.

What you need to be successful

Having covered the mistakes, a good question at this point is asking yourself what do you need to be successful? This is an extremely simple question to answer, thankfully.

It involves two things:

- Patience and dedication
- Understanding the basics

Patience and dedication

Rome was not built overnight, and neither will your strength and your body. On average, it takes about three months of constant training for you to see visible results in the mirror and for others to notice the changes in you. If you feel that three months is too far, then understand that there is no magic pill or procedure you can undergo that will immediately get you where you want to go. Life doesn't work that way.

Plus, three months isn't that long. You will spend your first month getting used to your routine, and the second month is where you will start connecting things together. By the third month, exercise will become a habit for you and you will start feeling the changes long before they appear in the mirror.

Things like the difference in how your clothes fit and your energy levels will make themselves known towards the end of the first month itself. The best way to look at your routine is to break it down into a series of small tasks. This way, you will avoid being overwhelmed and will be able to stick to your course better.

Understanding the basics

So how is strength built? How do your muscles grow? This process is much simpler than you can imagine. The amount of muscle mass in your body is referred to as lean body mass. The higher your lean body mass, the lower your body fat percentage. The higher your strength level, the greater your lean body mass.

So, it's pretty simple: the more muscle you have, the less body fat you carry and the stronger you are. When you exercise, your body is under stress. You may think that stress is a bad thing, but it's important to distinguish between the positive and negative versions of it.

Stress is terrible for us when it lasts for long periods of time. This is when your body starts producing hormones that disrupt your digestive system and put your brain on the edge, ready to fight back against any perceived threat (Stoppler, 2018). When it is present for short periods, stress is good for us as it forces us to grow and learn new skills.

This is pretty much what exercise does. If you try to exercise for hours on end, you will get hurt. An ideal workout lasts about an hour, followed by a nutritious meal within an hour of completion. Post-workout nutrition is important because, during your training session, your body breaks down muscle fibers.

During the post-workout nutrition and rest period, you will provide your body with the fuel it needs to repair itself and get stronger. Putting all of this together, the muscle building formula is pretty simple: focus on building strength, eat right, and rest well.

How this book will work for you

Each exercise presented in this book will lead you to build a base level of strength before moving up a notch. One of the best ways to keep your body from adapting to your current routine and to continually challenge itself is to keep adding new workouts aimed at increasing your strength level.

So, take the time to master a particular exercise before moving on to the next one. Don't be in a hurry to try everything at once as this will result in sabotaging yourself. Be patient and understand the basics. Review common mistakes and make sure you don't make them.

It sounds simple and it really is. The key to success is often as simple as avoiding complicating things unnecessarily.

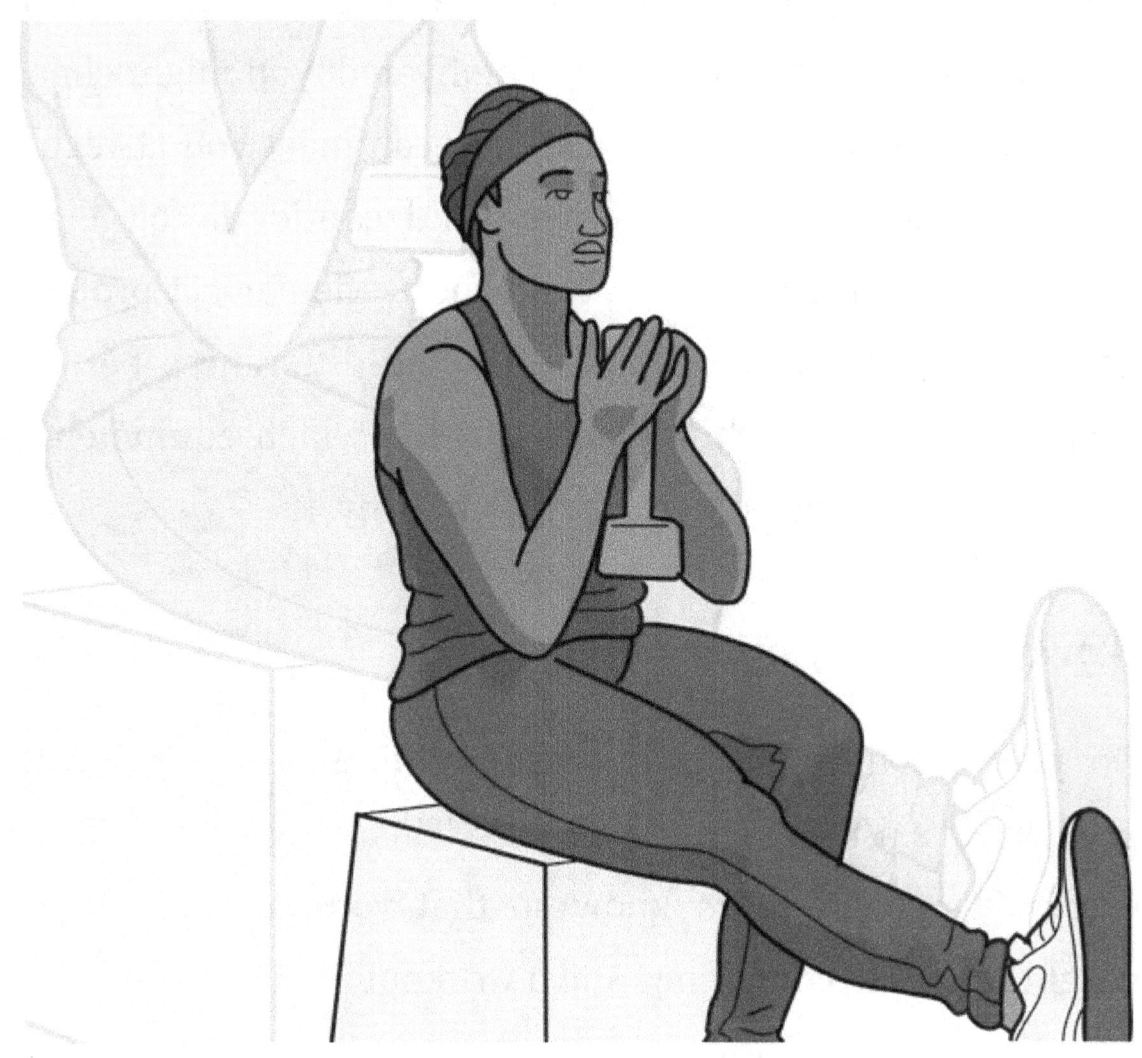

This chapter will focus on the issues to consider when evaluating the training environment and equipment options. Depending on your goals and schedule, you can opt for home workouts and need information on what you'll need at home to create your own gym. If you feel that a dedicated trainer and / or fitness space can help you stay motivated, you might choose to work out at a gym, where a trainer can meet you at regular times. To help you feel prepared and confident for a gym experience, we'll go over what to expect, the correct protocol, and clothing options. Do you know the differences between free weights and machines? We will see which equipment is best to help you with your schedule and why.

Workouts in the gym and at home

Do you feel intimidated by weight lifting at the gym? No problem, it's a normal feeling to try. This book will teach you everything you need to know so that you can walk to the weight rack with confidence and a workout plan in hand.

There are some fundamental differences between training in the gym and training at home. The first is the selection of equipment. The gym offers a large variety of weightlifting and cardio equipment, which is important as you progress through your schedule and need heavier weights. You will have multiple sets of dumbbells, kettlebells, barbells, resistance bands, cables and machines at your disposal. You'll also have access to heavier weights with safety mechanisms, such as a leg press machine and weight lifting rack where you can complete powerlifting movements. This type of equipment allows you to lift much heavier weights than you can at home due to the safety of the rack. It may seem too much to consider and it makes all of this feel intimidating, but all of these options are valuable because they give you more freedom to select what works best for you and your body. Another thing to consider about the gym is that there are instructors who can demonstrate proper use of the equipment and watch you to make sure you are using the equipment correctly.

The gym is also a great motivator because you have to make an effort and physically go there instead of staying in your home. Some people find that if they schedule time in the gym like other activities and aren't distracted at home, they are more likely to be consistent with their workouts. Also, when you are in the gym, you are close to other people and are more likely to work hard.

If after reading this book you still feel a little hesitant about lifting weights in the gym, take small steps. Start by grabbing some weights and find a corner at the gym to do your workout. If your gym has a studio for classes, the studio is a more private place to train when there isn't a class in session. If you are still unable to hit the gym, this book includes many tips for home workout hacks that will help you get the most out of your schedule while at home.

There are downsides to using a gym. Sometimes, there are lines to use the equipment, and you may have to wait for someone else to finish using a piece of equipment you want to use. Additionally, while most gyms are fairly clean, you may find that with continuous, non-stop use, some of the equipment's handles and seats need to be cleaned between uses. There is never a line for equipment at home, and everything is always clean and ready for use. But while a home gym may seem ideal, keep in mind that you will likely have less variety of equipment at your disposal and will need to keep buying heavier weights as you progress through your weightlifting program.

Whatever you choose, you need to find the best way to maximize your schedule. The most important thing is to commit to yourself and keep it no matter where you are.

The weights

There are basically two types of weights to consider: free weights and machines. Free weights are any type of weight that you can use freely in all planes of motion. Simply put, they're not attached to anything, so you have full control over them. The benefit of using free weights is that they are the most functional pieces of equipment, which means they allow you to move the same way you move in real life when going about your daily activities. Free weights help muscles develop under different stress lines, which is essential for injury prevention and better overall movement. You also need to be more careful with free weights because you have complete control over them. Therefore, there is nothing that will protect you if you use weights with the wrong shape. The machines are in fixed positions. You can only push or pull the weight in a particular stress line and in a particular movement. This is safer but not functional. You rarely do anything in real life that allows your body to move in a straight line along a single plane. This means that you could also put yourself at risk of injury when using a machine, because your anatomical structure and your natural way of moving may not be aligned with the machines.

All the exercises listed in the book will use free weights so that the exercises can be easily performed in the gym or home gym. Additionally, free weights allow exercise measurements to remain constant, which is important for tracking your progress. You need to know how much weight you are lifting at all times so that you can accurately track your progress. We will discuss the types of free weights used in this book in the following sections. Keep in mind that most of the exercises in this book can be done using either type of free weight.

DUMBBELLS

Dumbbells are short bars with weights at each end. The handlebars can be used individually or in pairs. This will allow you to work each arm independently of the other (or unilateral training). This is great for making sure one arm doesn't overcompensate the other and that your muscles are well balanced. Another benefit of using dumbbells is that you can position them in the way that best suits your joints, such as keeping them closer or further away from your body depending on what is comfortable for you. You can also rotate the handlebars internally and externally to adjust the comfort. Also, dumbbells are easier to drop if absolutely necessary while performing an exercise. You should never lower weights, especially as you transition from one exercise to another. However, if you don't have a spotter and have strained your muscles to failure, it is safer to drop weights than risk injury by holding on to dumbbells. If you have to drop the weights, always make sure you are in an open space and not hurting anyone else.

BALANCERS

Barbells, on the other hand, have a longer metal bar with weight discs on each end. Some barbells allow you to adjust the amount of weight on each end. Other barbells are a fixed weight, like with dumbbells. Barbells are great for loading when doing leg exercises. ("Loading" is a common term for adding more weight to a movement.) Since women tend to have more strength in the lower body than the upper body, it is easier to use heavier weights with barbells because the weight it is supported with the shoulders and upper back instead of just with the arms. Also, sometimes the barbells seem easier to use because you grab it with both hands; therefore, you are able to stabilize yourself better when performing pushing and pulling movements. On the downside, barbells can allow you to compensate by pushing harder with one side rather than the other, so be aware of this. Also, the barbells are a bit bulkier to have around the house and a little awkward to maneuver. Once you have learned how to use barbells, however, they are a great resource, especially for exercises where you want to use more weight. You can use dumbbells instead of barbells for exercises, but then you run the risk of losing your grip before completing the set. When this happens, you will probably need to put the dumbbells down before continuing the movement, which is not ideal. especially for exercises where you want to use heavier weight. You can use dumbbells instead of barbells for exercises, but then you run the risk of losing your grip before completing the set. When this happens, you will probably need to put the dumbbells down before continuing the movement, which is not ideal. especially for exercises where you want to use more weight. You can use dumbbells instead of barbells for exercises, but then you run the risk of losing your grip before completing the set. When this happens, you will probably need to put the dumbbells down before continuing the movement, which is not ideal. especially for exercises where you want to use more weight. You can use dumbbells instead of barbells for exercises, but then you run the risk of losing your grip before completing the set. When this happens, you will probably need to put the dumbbells down before continuing the movement, which is not ideal. especially for exercises where you want to use more weight. You can use dumbbells instead of barbells for exercises, but then you run the risk of losing your grip before completing the set. When this happens, you will probably need to put the dumbbells down before continuing the movement, which is not ideal.

GYM ETIQUETTE

Gym etiquette is very important if you want to maintain a positive gym environment. Nobody wants to raise with the woman who doesn't follow the rules. Don't be that woman! Here are some things to keep in mind.

Don't devour the equipment. Everyone is looking to get their workouts with limited equipment and time. Complete your set and then allow someone else to work with the equipment during the rest period. Sharing is the cure!

Clean up yourself. Just like sharing, other common kindergarten rules apply at the gym, including restoring the equipment to its original place. Detect weights and clean everything, including anything that may have come into contact with your sweat, such as benches, chairs, balls, handles, and cardio equipment.

Don't talk on the phone. Nobody wants to hear your latest gossip as they try to focus on their training. Bring your conversation to the lobby. Sending text messages is appropriate, but keep in mind how long you sit on the equipment while doing this. Two minutes is enough to rest. If there is something more, you should leave the car or the counter and let someone else use it.

Ask to work with someone. Don't just commandeer someone's weights or car without asking them. If you would like to use equipment someone else is using, please ask how many sets are left. Then wait for them to finish or ask to work (use weight or equipment while they rest) with them.

Practice good hygiene. Be sure to wear cool gym clothes and take proper measures to prevent odor once you start sweating by cooling your deodorant or antiperspirant before your workout. A good rule of thumb is that if you can smell yourself, others can probably smell you too. Also, carry a towel with you to remove excess sweat from yourself or the equipment you come in contact with. The gym is a much nicer place when everyone practices good hygiene.

Don't make it embarrassing for others. The gym is often filled with good-looking people with great bodies. However, they are there to train just like you. Be friendly, but remember to consider the gym more or less like a workplace, not a club.

Respect the training of others. It is perfectly fine to get inspired by training another member or a coach. However, don't copy everything someone else is doing in a workout. You don't know their goals and, if they are professionals, you are stealing their training. It is much nicer to go to the person when they are free and ask them if they would mind assisting you in creating some of your workouts. You can also ask them to explain the benefits of the exercise you were thinking of copying.

Clothing and other gear

Typically, women wear leggings or shorts to the gym to allow for dynamic movement. Sweatpants are fine too, although you may feel uncomfortable. Choose pants designed for training so that they are breathable and breathable to prevent discomfort or, worse, an infection. (Cotton underwear is also suggested for this reason.) Also wear a supportive sports bra and breathable top. You can choose a tank top or shirt with short or long sleeves, depending on your comfort level. Recommended fabrics for tops and bottoms include polyester, nylon, spandex, and cotton.

It is also recommended that you wear athletic sneakers. A sneaker designed for cross training would be best, as opposed to a running shoe or casual sneaker. You want the shoe to be supportive and relatively flat to allow for stability and dynamic movement when lifting weights. It's best to go to an athletics store and try a few different brands to find out what's best for you. Everyone's feet are different, so try on your first pair of sneakers and do some dynamic moves like walking, jumping, and squatting. You may also need insoles to correct any imbalances in your feet.

In terms of additional elements, there are a few things you should consider. Weight gloves are useful for preventing hands from developing calluses and for improving grip strength. It's also a good idea to have a bottle of water with you to stay hydrated during your workout, as well as a towel or two to wipe away sweat and lie down on common equipment. It is also helpful to carry a small drawstring bag with you to the gym to position all of these items to avoid cluttering the gym floor.

Creating a home gym

If you prefer to train at home rather than at the gym, I recommend that you purchase a set of dumbbells and a barbell to perform the training movements in this book. Look for a dumbbell set that allows you to change weight rather than a set with a fixed weight, this way you will only need one set instead of multiples. The same rule applies to buying a barbell - try to find one that allows you to add and remove discs in order to maximize your space. It's a good idea to buy iron dumbbells and barbells if you plan to keep the weights outside, as they hold up better in adverse weather conditions. You can get the colorful neoprene weights for indoor use.

If you have the space, a weight bench would also help. Other pieces of equipment to consider buying are a foam roller, stability ball, resistance bands, medicine ball, ankle weights, booty bands, a yoga mat, and a step. (You can purchase a kit of resistance bands that allow you to change handles, creating more resistance options. This is useful for saving space, similar to the tip above for dumbbells and barbells.) Decide what to buy based on what you feel is appropriate for your fitness level. All the equipment is very useful and will maximize your weight lifting experience at home. You can purchase any of these equipment online, which is great because it is delivered right to your front door.

When setting up your training space, choose a place with good lighting and a mirror if possible so you can check your form as you move. You want a lot of free space for dynamic movements, as you don't want to accidentally step on something or drop something. The mat is nice so it has extra padding for floor exercises; it's also a good way to muffle the noise when putting down weights. However, keep in mind that the carpet will be more unstable (which will make the movements more challenging) and it is more difficult to remove sweat from a carpet. I would recommend an easy-to-clean rubber floor installed specifically for your home gym. This type of flooring is stable, it has some elasticity to absorb the impact of more explosive movements and is easy to clean. Wooden floors are adequate.

Some people like to listen to music while they work out, so consider putting a stereo system in your home gym. It may also be useful to have a water source to refill the bottle during workouts. A portable fan or heater may also be needed to keep the gym at an ideal temperature while exercising.

All in all, the cost of a home gym depends on how much equipment you want and how much functional space you want to have. You can start with a simple $ 50 investment for a few pesos to get started. Investing in a full set of free weights could cost up to $ 500.

As you progress, you may want to invest in some cardio equipment for your home gym too. This could bring your cost closer to $ 2,000 in total. Start small with an initial investment and then add more equipment as your passion for weightlifting grows.

Chapter 8: The Foundations of a Healthy Life

While exercise is an integral part of a healthy lifestyle, it is only part of it. If nothing else, exercise is only half of it. This might seem surprising to you, but it is a fact (Carroll, 2015). There are three other things that are much more important to your health, and making sure they are in order will go a long way in good health.

In no particular order, these three things are:

1. **Water**
2. **To sleep**
3. **Diet**

This chapter will break down all of these three elements and by the end you will know exactly what you need to do for all of them. Let's start by looking at the water first.

Water

The old adage that you drink eight glasses of water a day is a useful metric for determining how much water you need to drink. However, keep in mind that this is general advice that isn't meant to suit everyone's needs. As you've probably learned so far, everyone is different.

About 60% of the human body is made up of water (Carroll, 2015). It is almost impossible to overestimate how vital water is to healthy functioning. Water affects our body's processes down to the cellular level, where it helps eliminate waste and invigorates us. Water also plays a significant role in the disposal of this waste through urine and sweat.

Speaking of sweat, water is what keeps your body temperature at healthy levels. If you get too hot, the sweat cools you and ensures you don't melt from the inside (Carroll, 2015). In addition to this, water also plays a vital role in lubricating the joints and cushioning them. Layers of water around your sensitive organs also protect them from damage.

These are just a few of the ways water helps your overall health. A major cause of ill health in the average American adult is dehydration. Dehydration occurs when you simply don't provide your body with enough water and your body will immediately let you know when this occurs.

Some of the symptoms of dehydration are:

- Headache

- Lack of energy

- Inability to focus on tasks

- Tiredness or exhaustion

There are a few factors that determine the amount of water you need to drink each day. While the eight drink recommendation is a good place to start, depending on certain factors, you may find that you need to drink a lot more.

Ideal quantity

To understand how much water you need to drink, we need to take a look at the factors that affect the fluid levels in your body. The first and most obvious factor to consider is the climate you live in. Adult males living in temperate or pleasant climates require about 16 cups (four liters) of water, while adult females require 12 cups (three liters) per day.

The warmer the climate you live in, the more you'll sweat and need to replenish the fluid you've lost. There is no way to calculate this accurately, but it is always better to increase the frequency with which you drink the water the hotter it gets. The next factor that affects fluid intake is exercise.

The more you train, the more you sweat, and therefore your need for water is greater. It's a good idea to drink some water before your workout as this will give you energy and ensure you don't get dehydrated in the middle of your workout. In between exercises, get into the habit of sipping some water. Once you're done, take a big swig of water while you rest and get ready to consume your post-workout meal.

I recommend sticking to plain water instead of consuming fancy sports drinks. These drinks have their uses for people who train for periods lasting more than a couple of hours. When you exercise for that long, your body will lose electrolytes and these drinks can help replenish them. However, for the purposes of the exercise program in this book, you don't need it.

Avoid consuming high-caffeinated drinks before your workout as they dehydrate you to a greater extent than regular drinks. They will give you a nice boost of energy, but unless you work out first thing in the morning, you don't need that stimulation.

Finally, pregnant or nursing women should increase their fluid intake by at least two cups from the recommended intake amounts mentioned earlier (Gunnars, 2018). Check yourself for signs of dehydration and consult your doctor at all times.

How to consume

You can consume water in several ways. First of all, there is drinking, which is the most obvious way to do it. You can drink water or fluids, other than heavily caffeinated drinks. To clarify, these drinks contain water, but their calories come at a cost as you will learn shortly. Don't consume them in excess.

Beverages like milkshakes, smoothies or juices contain copious amounts of water. If you are a juicer enthusiast, you can consume vegetable juices that contain high levels of water, such as green leafy vegetables or cucumbers. Drinking fruit juices, such as watermelon, is also a great way to get your daily allowance of water.

Develop a routine around drinking water. Personally, I use a 40-ounce bottle to make sure I'm drinking the right amount of water every day. I fill the flask at least three times, so I know I'm drinking at least 120 ounces a day (roughly just under a liter of water). You can continue sipping from your bottle throughout the day and monitoring yourself for signs of inadequate fluid intake.

The signs to watch out for are (Gunnars, 2018):

- Constantly feeling thirsty or hungry
- The urine is yellow in color or not colorless

Thirst is sometimes confused as hunger, so always drink some water when you're hungry just to make sure you don't cross the strings. All in all, with a little discipline, you can make sure you don't have to worry about your water intake throughout the day.

Too much water?

Is it possible to drink too much water? Technically yes. Excessive water consumption leads to a condition called hyponatremia (Gunnars, 2018). This occurs when the blood is highly diluted to the extent that its sodium content is too low. Under such conditions, your kidneys cannot excrete excess water.

Athletes who train for long periods of time are subject to it. In general, it is difficult for the average American adult to achieve such levels of risk, so you probably don't need to worry about that.

To sleep

I have already mentioned in the previous chapter how vital the recovery period is to your progress. In fact, your gains are not achieved during training but during the rest period. The most significant factor affecting the quality of your recovery is sleep. To be more precise, the quality of it.

Just like with water, the average adult requires at least eight hours of sleep every 24 hours (Roland, 2019). There are some exceptions of people who manage to get by on only six hours of sleep, but these people are very rare. If you think you are one of them, chances are you are underestimating your need for sleep.

The fact is, the average adult carries a significant sleep deficit. This is due to a variety of lifestyle factors. Additionally, the type of lifestyle you lead also determines how much sleep you need. Some people actually take longer than the normal eight hours. Let's take a look at what happens when we sleep before trying to figure out how much is needed.

Eat high quality protein to increase strength gains

The sixth and final strategy for unlocking your fitness potential is to eat high quality protein with each meal to increase strength gains. Protein in your diet is the raw material for building muscle mass and strength.

The importance of eating enough high quality protein cannot be underestimated. Performing strength exercises with insufficient protein intake hinders muscle development.

Research shows that it is more difficult to reverse age-related muscle loss and improve strength in the elderly if they do not have adequate protein intake. Studies have also shown that older adults need more protein than their younger counterparts. Inadequate protein intake is a concern for seniors and not only contributes to muscle loss but also results in increased skin fragility, reduced immune system function, poorer healing and longer recovery times after the illness. A review published in Current Opinion in Clinical Nutrition and

Metabolic Care recommended seniors to consume 25-30 grams of high-quality protein per meal to improve muscle growth and prevent age-related muscle loss.

What makes protein "high quality"?

It's a combination of three things:

1. **How easily your body can break down proteins into its parts (called amino acids).**

2. **The actual parts a protein will become when your body breaks it down (its amino acid profile).**

3. **How much parts are available to support muscle maintenance and growth.**

High-quality protein is easily broken down by your body, contains all the parts your body needs to build muscle, and is readily available for your body to use. Not all sources of protein contain all of the building blocks your body needs to build muscle. For example, many vegetables contain protein, but they are of low quality.

The following foods contain high quality proteins that provide everything your body needs.

Remember, the goal is to consume 25-30 grams of protein per meal:

<u>Animal</u>

- Chicken breast (3 ounces): 28 grams of protein
- Steak (3 ounces): 26 grams of protein
- Turkey (3 ounces): 25 grams of protein
- Lamb (3 ounces): 23 grams of protein
- Pork (3 ounces): 22 grams of protein
- Egg (large): 8 grams of protein

<u>Seafood</u>

- Salmon (3 ounces): 22 grams of protein
- Tuna (3 ounces): 22 grams of protein
- Tilapia (3 ounces): 22 grams of protein
- Cod (3 ounces): 20 grams of protein
- Rainbow trout (3 ounces): 20 grams of protein
- Shrimp (3 ounces): 20 grams of protein

Dairy

- Greek yogurt (6 ounces): 18 grams of protein
- Cottage cheese (4 ounces): 14 grams of protein
- Regular yogurt (1 cup): 11 grams of protein
- Milk (1 cup): 8 grams of protein
- Mozzarella (1 ounce): 7 grams of protein

Vegetarian / vegan

- Pinto beans and rice blend (1 cup): 11 grams of protein
- Black bean and rice blend (1 cup): 8 grams of protein
- Tofu (3.5 ounces): 8 grams of protein
- Soy milk (1 cup): 8 grams of protein

When it comes to maintaining and building muscle mass and strength, eating enough high-quality protein is just as important as doing strength exercises regularly. But before making any changes to your diet, be sure to speak to your doctor.

Key points

- Protein in your diet is the raw material for building muscle mass and strength. It is more difficult to reverse aging-related muscle loss and improve strength in the elderly without adequate protein intake.

- In addition to performing strength exercises regularly, seniors should consume 25-30 grams of high-quality protein with each meal to enhance muscle growth and prevent age-related muscle loss.

Stages of action

- Use the high-quality protein list provided in this chapter to get an idea of how much protein you are consuming at each meal. Do you eat 25-30 grams of high quality protein each time? If not, what changes can be made?

- If you are a family member or career for an older adult who would like to help with exercise, use the list to get an idea of how much protein they are consuming at each meal. Is it 25-30 grams? If not, what changes can be made?

In Part 2, you learned seven strategies to unlock your fitness potential. If you follow each one exactly, I guarantee you will experience noticeable improvements in your strength, balance and energy in two short weeks.

Stages of sleep

Sleep is often considered a passive or inactive state. After all, all you have to do is lie there like a log and keep your eyes closed while your brain and body take care of everything else. While your body is at rest, the same is not true of your brain. If nothing else, it's just as active as it is when you're awake. The difference is that the processes it performs differ depending on what stage of sleep you are in.

There are two major stages of sleep: non-REM and REM. REM stands for Rapid Eye Movement. When you go to bed for bed, you enter the non-REM phase, which is divided into three phases. The first phase lasts about 10 minutes and is characterized by light sleep and at this time you can be easily awakened.

The second phase of non-REM sleep lasts nearly 30 minutes and is when you drift deeper into sleep. You may be awakened at this stage, but it is a little harder to do so. The final phase is the longest one and lasts about 40 minutes. This is when your brain finally decides it's the right time to start doing what it needs to do. Your blood pressure drops, as does your heart rate, and you start getting into REM sleep.

REM, as the name suggests, is characterized by eye movements under the eyelids. While in non-REM mode, your brain slows things down, but here it picks up the pace (Roland, 2019). Your heart rate and body temperature increase as your brain starts processing things that happened throughout the day and begins to incorporate any new skills you've learned.

Essentially, this is the period when your brain forms new neural pathways and makes connections within it. Research suggests that REM sleep is primarily concerned with restoring the brain and not so much the body (Roland, 2019).

When you sleep, you drift between periods of REM and non-REM sleep. After the first period of REM sleep, you will not return to the first phase of non-REM sleep, but you will remain suspended around the second stage. This is why loud noises in the middle of the night can wake you up. Physical repair occurs during the non-REM phase.

This is when human growth hormone or HGH is secreted, which is used to repair muscles and other soft tissues that have been subjected to stress during exercise. HGH is responsible for muscle growth and the only time it is present in the body in large quantities is during non-REM sleep. So, skip sleep and are not giving your body a chance to recover as needed.

Quality

It is tempting to think of sleep in terms of quantity and to think that as long as you enter the hours, everything is fine. This is a mistake. It's a bit like thinking that being in the gym doing nothing will cause muscle growth. There are a number of things that affect the quality of your sleep. The recommendation to sleep for eight hours assumes that those eight hours are of high quality.

If you exercise regularly or lead an active lifestyle, you need more than eight hours of sleep. The exact amount isn't known, but a great way to get the ideal amount of sleep is to simply go to bed without setting the alarm. Wake up whenever your body wants the next day. If you need to wake up at a specific time, taking naps during the day is a great way to increase productivity (Roland, 2019).

Ensuring total darkness in your bedroom and developing a sleep routine is essential for getting quality sleep. Limit the time you stare at a bright screen like your smartphone or TV. Your brain will process the large amount of light as a signal to stay awake. Read a book while you lie down to start preparing your brain for sleep.

While white noise (regular, rhythmic noise at a low pitch) can help produce good quality sleep, you want to limit erratic noise as this has been shown to reduce sleep quality (Roland, 2019). You should make sure that the bedding and pillows are also of good quality.

Deficit

The reality of our busy schedules often makes it impossible to always guarantee a high quality sleep. This does not mean that you should give up hope of a good sleep. One way to still get the hours you need is to take naps during the day. These naps can last up to 30 minutes and will make you feel refreshed. It will also help you avoid the mid-afternoon fog that hits people around 2:30 pm-3pm.

Another way is to go to bed on weekends (or whenever you have a day off) without setting the alarm. Let your body and brain decide how much sleep you need. If you feel the need to sleep all day, so be it. It is not possible to completely overcome a large sleep deficit. What I mean is you can't accumulate a month of lost sleep and then try to make up for it over the course of a week by not setting the alarm.

To overcome this deficit, you will need to follow good sleep habits and make sure you develop a routine that will ensure you get the highest quality sleep possible. Finally, develop some consistency around your sleep habits. In other words, go to bed and wake up at the same time every day. Your body will get used to this and will automatically start shutting down during these times.

If you haven't slept well during the night, get up at the same time to maintain consistency and try to catch up on lost sleep over the weekend. Prioritize sleep and you will find that many of your fatigue and lethargy problems will disappear.

Diet

When it comes to losing fat and staying healthy, exercise is essential, but above all it is diet that plays the most significant role. In fact, it is possible to lose fat without exercising, although I don't recommend this approach for the sake of your overall health.

If you think the fitness industry produces material that confuses people, that's nothing compared to what the diet industry does. There are all kinds of fancy diets out there that restrict one form of food and promote the other. These work on various levels. To be sure, most of them are legitimate. This is mainly because healthy eating isn't rocket science.

Our bodies have an intuitive knowledge of what it needs to feed itself. The problem is that we complicate eating too much to the point that we end up getting confused. The following tips will help you make sure you eat clean and maintain a healthy diet.

Choose Fresh

Always choose fresh, whole foods over refined and processed foods. More than anything, this will go a long way in making sure you are eating healthily. Whole food refers to what exists in its natural form and is consumed with some cooking. Examples of whole foods include grains, vegetables, meat, fruit, and so on. There is a school of thought that advocates the consumption of food in a form that is closer to its natural state. This is generally good advice to follow, but there's no need to get fanatic about it.

Processed food can be a bit of a mess to make you dizzy at first. Technically speaking, everything that is not present in nature is processed. For example, wine is processed, as is cheese. In moderate quantities, they are not harmful. The types of processed foods you want to avoid at all costs are those that are chemically manipulated.

The food industry makes more money by producing things that last longer.

To ensure this, they add chemicals and sugar that achieve this. The problem is these chemicals wreak havoc on our internal organs and disrupt our digestive system. Anything that comes in a box, such as frozen pizza, fast food, TV dinners and so on, should be avoided.

Meat and oil are the two foods that most undergo processing. With meat, processing usually takes place in the type of feed provided to the animal and in the conditions in which it is housed. It goes without saying that most of the supermarket meat comes from farms that follow horrible practices (Myers, 2016). In some cases, livestock are fed plastic and other unnatural feed which results in all sorts of diseases that are transferred to you when you consume them.

The oil is processed to ensure better cooking. A telltale sign of processed oil is its color. Cold pressed natural oil such as coconut or extra virgin olive oil is not light in color or tends to freeze quickly. Furthermore, they tend to be viscous. Processed oils have an almost watery consistency and are light in color.

Chemicals are added during the extraction process to squeeze the last few bits of oil from the skins of whatever oil is taken. For example, olive oil itself can be processed, which is why it is best to stick to extra virgin olive oil, as opposed to olive pomace oil, which is chemically processed.

Choose the right sugar

In addition to meat and oil, sugar is available in processed and unprocessed forms. Processed sugar is generally bad for you and is responsible for most of the fat gains. Natural sugar, such as that found in fruit, honey, and even whole grains, are natural carbohydrates and are important for nutrition.

Choose natural sugar as much as possible. That said, remember that too much of anything is bad. Just because natural sugar is good for you doesn't mean you can drink honey all day instead of water. Make sure your diet is balanced. Choosing whole grains and fresh fruit in your diet is the best way to make sure you are getting the right amounts of this.

Eat protein

Your muscles are literally made of protein, and the fact is that the average American diet is high in carbohydrates and severely lacking in protein. A good rule of thumb is to eat 0.7-1 grams of protein per pound of body weight. So, if you weigh 200 pounds, you need to eat between 140 and 200 grams of protein as part of your diet.

There are a number of healthy sources of protein, both animal and plant. Animal sources tend to be denser and contain a higher concentration of protein within them. Plant sources usually contain a higher level of carbohydrates along with proteins. This is not bad in any way. It's just that you may need to train at higher intensity levels to burn off excess carbohydrates.

Monitor salt and sugar

I've already mentioned sugar, but salt is something most people ignore. Either they consume too little or they eat too much. Crowds who eat too much usually end up eating processed food, which appears to be high in sodium (i.e. salt).

It's easy to overeat by simply forgetting to add salt to the food you cook or not adding enough.

There is no need to think about it too much. Add a few pinches of salt and check how much water your body is holding. If you find that your stomach is full of water and you are constantly thirsty, you are probably eating too much salt (as long as you are not dehydrated).

As for sugar, it's possible to eat too much of the right kind of sugar. Any excess carbohydrate or sugar your body receives tends to convert into fat, so you need to make sure you limit your consumption.

Break up your meals

This is a controversial topic, but for starters it's best to eat smaller meals throughout the day. This is because it keeps your blood sugar levels constant and you will avoid experiencing the hunger spikes that occur when your blood sugar levels drop. Be careful, though: it can be easy to overeat when you do. Adjust meal portions in advance to minimize this risk.

See what you drink

When planning your meals, it's easy to measure how much you eat, but most people forget to keep track of how much they drink. A cup of coffee here and a juice there add up over the course of the day, and you can easily consume over 500 calories this way. It's best to stick to plain water if you want to have a drink.

If you drink coffee, minimize the milk and sugar you add or, even better, limit yourself to herbal teas or green tea. Processed beverages like Coke and other assorted carbonated drinks only make matters worse. It goes without saying that alcohol of any kind guarantees that you will consume more calories than necessary.

I'm not saying you should get rid of these things. Just minimize them while acknowledging that deletion is the best option.

Exercise

We all routinely eat more calories than we need. The best way to ensure we stay fit is to be physically active. Your bodyweight training routine will go a long way to ensure this, but try to be as active as possible. This means walking short distances instead of driving them. When you can, take the stairs instead of using the elevator.

Don't think of this as a routine. Make physical activity a part of your daily life and you will find yourself burning calories naturally. Also, exercise makes you hungry, which is a sign that your body is burning what you give it efficiently.

Meal Prep

How would you like a method that ensures you always eat the right food in the right quantities? Meal preparation is your answer! How you choose to prepare will be different from what someone else may decide to do. After all, your schedule determines how you will do this.

Many elements go into good meal preparation, so let's go through them one by one.

Storage

Understanding how to store food should be your first step. This is easy enough to do. You can purchase plastic containers or glass bowls that you can use for this purpose. Storing food in plastic is not a great idea in the long run as food will interact with it and produce harmful chemicals (Zandonella, 2010).

Storing food in glasses is best due to the lack of harmful by-products and the fact that you can safely reheat the food in the bowl itself. In addition to this, you also want to refer to the U.S. Department of Agriculture guidelines on food storage safety. As a general rule, don't aim to store food for more than three days in the refrigerator.

This means your cooking program is easy to understand.

Cooking program

If you store food for three days maximum in your refrigerator, it means that you will be cooking twice a week. Although the three-day rule applies to many foods, there are some items you can store longer, such as chopped vegetables, cooked beans, and so on.

A twice a week cooking schedule means you'll cook once on the weekend and once during the week. The weekday cooking session will need to be done efficiently if your schedule is full. This is why it is a good idea to cook or cook food slowly. Take your time to create imaginative dishes and recipes over the weekend.

I'm not saying your cooked weekday meals need to be flavorless. It is entirely possible to cook food quickly and easily and still keep it great. It's just a matter of learning to cook.

Your tools

If you have limited time to cook, one of the best things you can do is focus on cooking or slow cooking your dishes. This allows you to toss the food into the appliance and do something else while it cooks. The best part about this is that almost any type of food can be cooked this way. You can cook or slow cook meat, vegetables, grains, etc.

Make sure you have the right tools for preparing food. This means having good quality knives, baking sheets and sheets, and a food processor. I recommend a food processor rather than a blender as this will allow you to do more than just a blender.

Use smart recipes

Understand that the taste of your dish and the time it takes to create it have nothing to do with each other. A simple five-ingredient recipe that takes just 10 minutes to assemble can be as delicious as a recipe that has 20 ingredients and takes two hours to cook.

A great way to cut down on cooking times is to have smoothies or juices. This is especially true during breakfast. A good life hack is to add cocoa powder to any smoothie whose ingredients aren't palatable to you. You can throw in some protein like eggs, milk, veggies, avocado, peanut butter, or whatever strikes you and have a ready breakfast in no time.

If you feel hungry between meals, consider carrying around a mix of traces or assorted nuts. These are high in calories and will keep you full with a little help. Focus on creating recipes that require simple baking or baking and no longer require cooking methods to combine.

Salads are really easy to put together in general. You can prepare the ingredients in advance and store them in the refrigerator. If you are adding meat, you can choose to only cook this part of the recipe before consuming the meal.

Maintain balance

The best way to create balanced meals is to ensure a variety of textures and colors on the plate. It seems absurd to suggest color diversity, but this is one of the best ways to ensure you are eating a balanced meal. A simple formula of grains + proteins + veggies followed by a fruit-based snack or dessert almost always works.

Make sure you have a small serving of veggies with your meals and you'll tick almost all the boxes.

Meal preparation doesn't have to be complicated. With a little planning and prioritization, you'll make sure your meals are tasty, delicious, and healthy.

Chapter 9: Workout knowledge about body weight: warming up, stretching and breathing correctly

Now that we've covered some lifestyle basics, it's time to delve into the basics of bodyweight exercise. The good news is you don't need any form of equipment other than a pull-up bar. This is optional too as what you basically need is a sturdy platform to hang on and pull yourself up. As you progress into more advanced rhythmic gymnastics, you will need some equipment, but for now a pull-up bar is more than enough.

The rest of this chapter will give you everything you need to know about breathing, progression, rate, and so on.

Training frequency and other concerns

In the beginning, you should train three times a week with a one-day interval between workouts, as previously mentioned. This is to give your body enough time to recover and also gives you the mental space to adjust to your workouts. Remember, the best types of training are those that are as repeatable as possible.

If you were to stubbornly rush into a new workout routine, your brain and body would rebel at the sudden change. Habit is a powerful thing, and if you're not used to working out, your body simply won't accept the new changes to its routine, no matter how excited or motivated you are.

Very soon, you'll find yourself getting lazy or developing mysterious `` injuries " that will cause you to miss out on workouts, and sure enough, you'll be back to sitting on your couch in no time. Stick to the above schedule and you'll be fine. At first you may find it extremely easy and you may not feel the "sting" of a workout. This is intentional and allows your body to slowly get used to the new routine.

Where to start

The chapters following this will list the exercises you will need to perform. Each chapter will begin by describing the simplest form of the exercise and then proceed to more challenging forms. Each comes with different levels of strength, so it can be difficult to understand where exactly you need to start.

A good rule of thumb is to try all versions of an exercise. When you find that you can do about four repetitions of an exercise variation, start by doing the exercise that is one step lower. For example, the next chapter is entirely devoted to pushups and the progression is as follows:

- Knee pushup
- Inclined flexion
- Lift
- Diamond / Archer / Incline one arm Pushup
- One-arm pushup
- Weighted pushup

Let's say you can do four push-ups. This means that your starting level will be the knee pushup. To begin with, you should do three sets of four repetitions of knee pushups. Performing four reps of the knee pushup counts as one set. You will perform one set, rest, then perform another and so on until three sets are completed.

Rest periods

How long should you rest between sets? Aim for an average rest period of one minute with up to two minutes. Despite the average word, don't rest for 30 seconds after the first set and one minute and thirty seconds after the second set. Keep your rest periods consistent and you will see progress. Do not rest for more than two minutes.

If you feel the need to do this, you are probably progressing too fast and need to take things down one level.

Progression

As you begin, you will perform three sets of four repetitions per exercise variation. After the first day, you will rest for a day. In the next session, try to increase the first set by a single rep while keeping the same number of reps remaining. For example, your pushup progression will look like the one below:

Training day no. 1 - push-ups on the knees (4,4,4)

Day of rest

Training day no. 2 - push-ups on the knees (5,4,4)

Day of rest

Training day # 3 - push-ups on the knees (5,5,4)

Day of rest

Training day # 4 - push-ups on the knees (5,5,5)

Day of rest

Training day # 5 - push-ups on the knees (6,5,5)

And so on. You should aim to do three sets of eight reps with each variation before moving on to the next level. Following our push-up example, once you can do (8,8,8) of the knee bend, your next workout will be to do the push-up for (3,3,3). Try to increase the reps in the same way.

Don't try to shorten this process by adding more than one repetition for the reasons mentioned above regarding how your body adjusts to your new routine. Take it easy and you will find yourself making more progress in the long run.

Shortcuts

I'll keep this simple: there aren't any. Each repetition should be done throughout the full range of motion without trying to reduce progress. Any repetition that you cannot perform with the full range of motion does not count as a valid rep. Do not take a 10 second break between sets to perform the last rep. Keep your cadence as consistent as possible.

Cadence

Speaking of cadence, you should dedicate two seconds to the concentric phase and three seconds to the eccentric phase. Concentric phases are when you tense your muscles, while eccentric is when you release the pressure. In a pushup, the concentric phase is when you come down to the floor, and the eccentric phase is when you walk away from the floor (Cross, 2018).

You should pause for about a second between phases.

Stall

With this program, stalling shouldn't be a major concern. If you follow the progression as outlined, you will find that going from (8,8,8) to (4,4,4) of the highest level should come easily. Sometimes, it is possible that the next level is too difficult and you cannot complete (4,4,4). In these cases, increase the number of repetitions in the progression below 12 and try again.

In other words, if you find that you are unable to complete (4,4,4), go down one level and aim to increase your reps to (12,12,12) from (8,8,8.) This will generally solve all problems.

If you are still unable to complete (4,4,4) of the highest progression, aim for (3,3,3) and start there.

Another form of stall that occurs is within the current level itself. For example, you may not be able to progress beyond (7,7,7) for any reason. Lack of progress from a single session doesn't count as a stall. If you are unable to progress beyond three sessions, eliminate the number of reps you are doing.

This means that you will perform (6,6,6) during the next session and then go back up to (7,7,7). This applies to all combinations of repetitions. For example, if you were stuck on (7,7,6), you will still load at (6,6,6) and go back. Another good idea is to monitor your rest and recovery periods. You want to feel fresh and ready to start training. If you're exhausted just thinking about it, take another day off and come back refreshed.

Imbalances

Eventually you will move on to variations of one arm exercise and these will present a challenge. Almost everyone has some form of strength imbalance and you will find that you will be able to do more reps on one side rather than the other. To eliminate it, start with the weak side first and do the same number of reps on the stronger side, although you can do more.

Warm ups

A good workout routine starts with a great warm-up. As I mentioned above, warming up is something we naturally understand and yet fail to implement when it comes to exercise. I'm not sure what the reasons for this are, and it's not important to delve into everything. Suffice it to say that you should warm up whatever happens.

Excellent warm-up reduces the risk of injury by warming the body temperature to a certain extent (Cross, 2018). Warm muscles are more flexible and respond better to stimulation. In practical terms, this means that you will perform better and have a reduction in pain after training.

Pain is something you will have to deal with in the beginning as your body is not used to the activity you are putting it through. This makes it even more important for you to prepare your body before a workout. A good warm-up ensures that your body is prepared for the more strenuous movement that it has to follow and also mentally prepares you for your workout.

So with that said, let's take a look at the best warm-up routine you should implement before your workouts.

Step # 1: Jump or jump rope

Skipping a rope has long been used as an effective warm-up not only by bodybuilders but also by athletes and boxers. It gets the blood flowing and also helps with coordination. If you can't jump a rope to save your life, you can jump in the same spot, run in the same spot, or do jumping jacks.

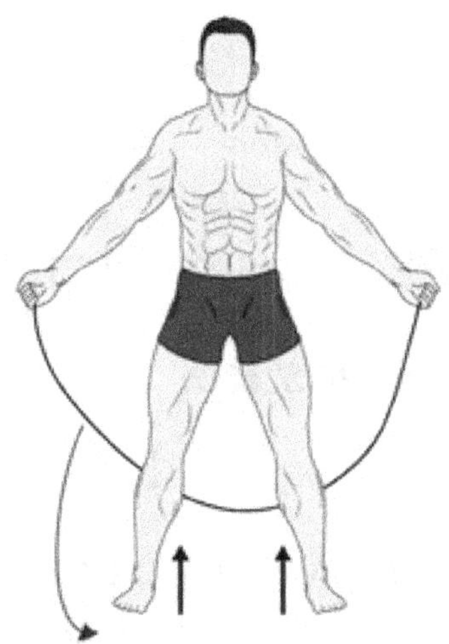

Run in place or jump rope for 5 minutes.

Step # 2 - Shoulder rotations

Opening the joints is extremely important and the shoulder rotations do the job admirably. The exercise is pretty simple. Simply rotate both arms back in a controlled manner. You can also move them forward if that's more comfortable for you. Alternatively, you can do one arm at a time.

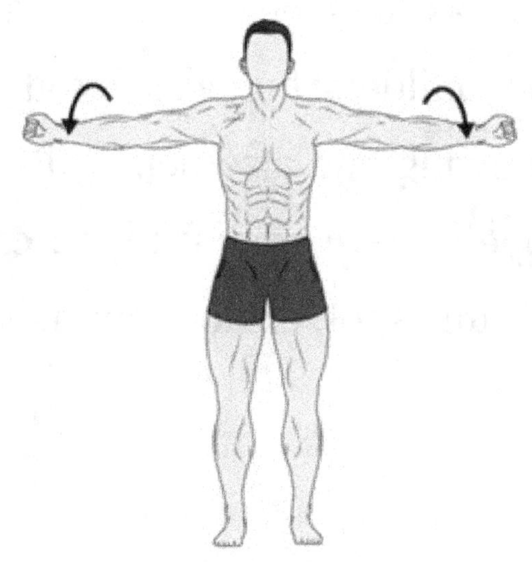

Perform 5 shoulder rotations per arm.

Step # 3 - The arm goes up

This exercise also focuses on loosening the shoulder joints. Just raise your arms above your head and swing them up and down in a controlled manner. You don't want to wield your power here as you swing. Just focus on how the shoulder moves and focus on the increased sense of warmth as the blood flows through it.

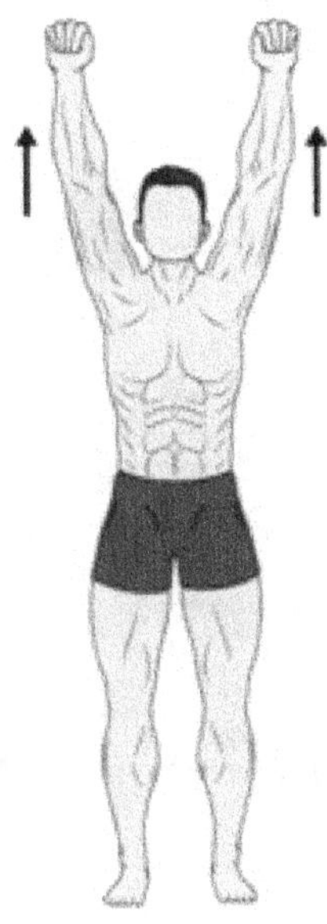

Do 5 arm raises for both arms.

Step # 4 - Torso twists

From the shoulders, now let's move on to the hips. Rotate your core left and right in a controlled manner. As you turn around, notice how your lower back feels. You can try to tighten your core when you reach the end of your twist.

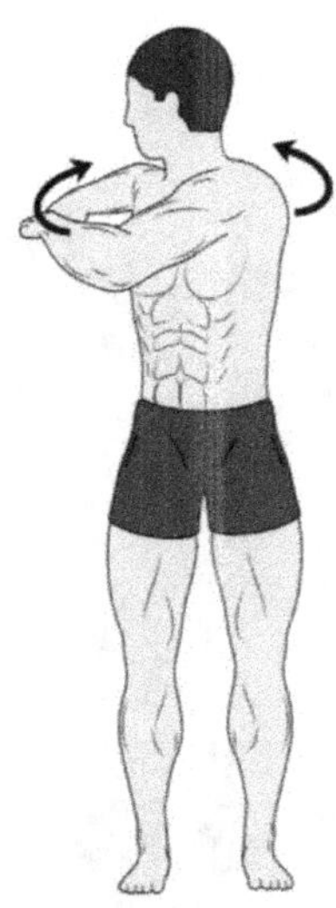

Do 5 torso twists. Remember that a twist left and right counts as a single twist.

Step # 5: chest expansion

The chest is one of the largest muscles in the body and is more of a muscle chain than a single muscle. It practically encompasses the entire upper body, so loosening it up is essential if you want to perform your workout well. Put your arms by your side; bring them up and out as you expand your chest.

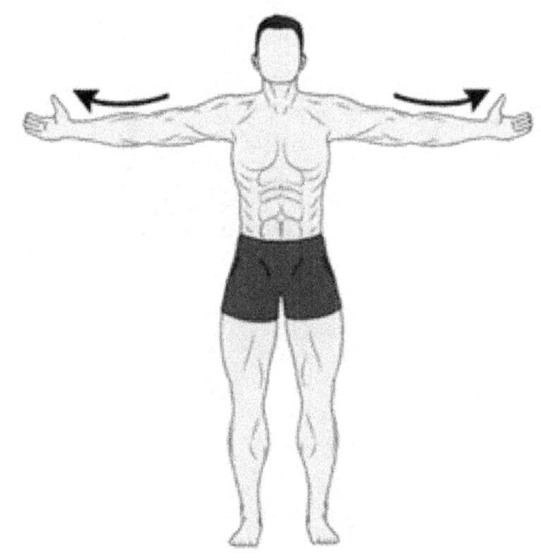

Do 5 chest expansions with palms facing up.

Step # 6 - Neck rotations

Your neck contains important muscles that stabilize your head. During training, these muscles receive automatic training, and if they are not warmed up properly, they can cause sprains and other unwanted things. Simply rotate your head clockwise or counterclockwise.

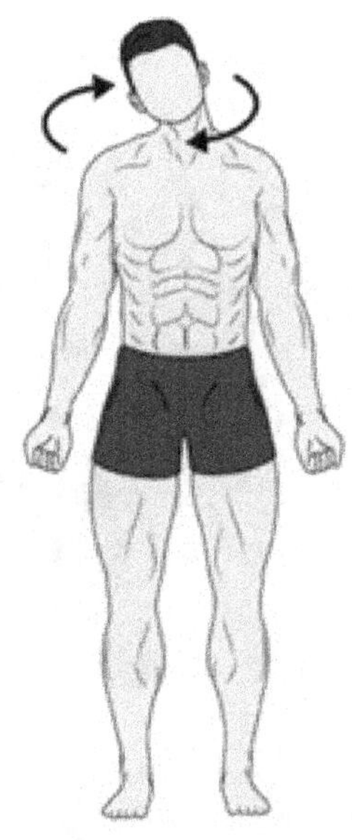

Do 5 left and 5 right.

Step # 7 - Hip rotation

Thanks to sitting all day, your hips are likely locked. The hip joint is one of the most flexible in the body and has a wide range of motion. This exercise unlocks it. Adopt a staggering stance, just like a boxer would. Lift your back leg off the ground and rotate your hip to bring it forward. This is a single rotation.

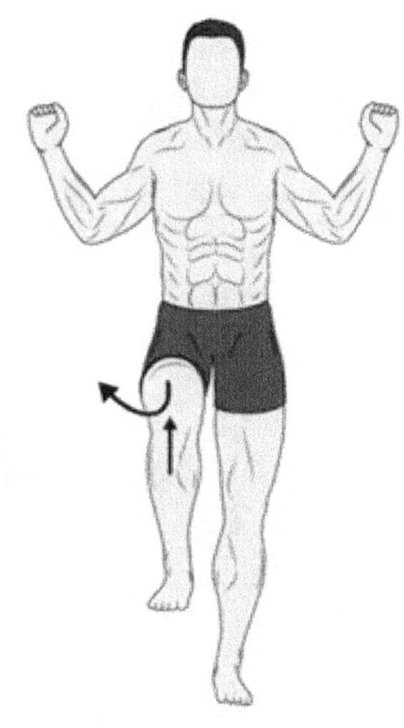

Perform 5 hip rotations on each leg.

Step # 8: Reverse Hip Rotation

Once you have finished the previous exercise, rotate your hips in the opposite direction from the same position. In the previous exercise, you brought your leg forward. Now turn your hip back to loosen them even more.

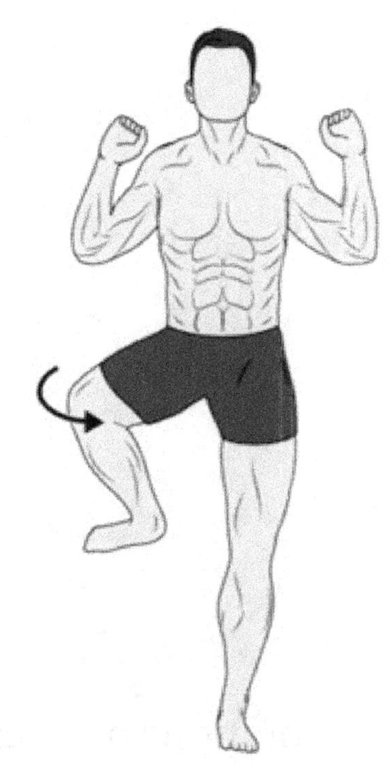

Perform 5 reverse hip rotations on each leg.

Step # 9 - Leg Swing

From a standing position, place your right arm in front of you. Now, lift your right leg forward until you reach the level of the extended arm. Raise your leg in a controlled manner. This is a raise and not a kick. That said, you don't need to lift it too slowly. Experiment with which speed works best for you and focus on loosening your hips and hamstrings.

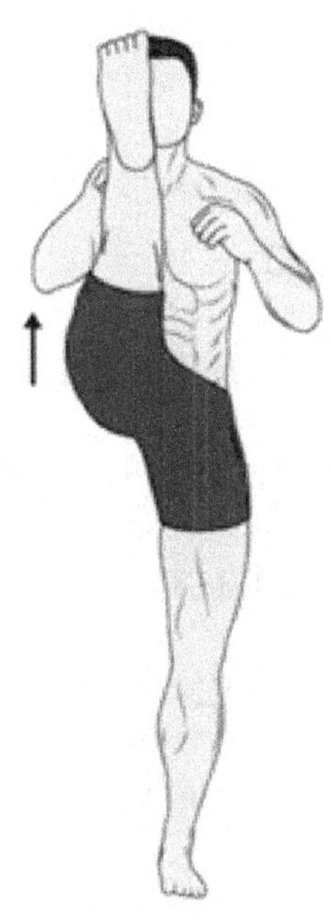

Do 5 leg swings per leg.

Loosening your hips is extremely important, and if you feel they haven't warmed up properly yet, you can do a couple of variations of the leg swing. Hold on to a vertical frame of some kind at arm's length and stand next to it. Your arm will then be extended at your side. Swing the leg furthest from the frame back and forth. Repeat with the other leg.

Now face the frame and place both hands on it, with your torso bent at an angle of about 60 degrees. Swing your left leg from side to side while keeping your torso as straight as possible. Repeat with the right leg.

Post workout routine

Don't be alarmed by reading the name of this section. There are no additional exercises to perform once you are done. Instead, you'll need to start stretching after your workout to start the recovery process. Many people ignore this part of their training, including experienced trainees.

The fact is, post-workout stretches play an essential role in recovery. You will be less sore in the following days and will feel more relaxed once finished. Let's take a look at some of the benefits of an excellent post-workout stretching routine.

Flexibility

Strength is not only measured by the amount of muscle you have, but also by how flexible that muscle is. While mass generates power, flexibility is what ensures that the muscle is flexible and does not sag when stressed in unusual ways. During the workout, your muscles will be grouped to generate power.

Loosening them improves flexibility and also improves performance for your next workout by improving the recovery process.

Blood circulation

When a muscle stiffens, the blood flow within it narrows. Other than that, your heart will pump at a faster rate and your body overall is very stressed. Stretching while cooling down improves blood circulation. Recovery begins when oxygen-rich blood begins to flow through the muscles. This allows the muscle tissue cells to repair themselves and become stronger.

Lactic acid

When your muscles are stressed, the oxygen within them runs out as your body will use up all the oxygen it can get its hands on. This leads to the formation of lactic acid, which gradually increases as you train. One of the things that increases the rate of lactic acid dissipation is the increase in blood flow.

Stretching achieves this by improving blood flow through the muscles and hence the damage caused by lactic acid production is significantly reduced.

Energy boost

When your body cools down, your brain releases endorphins. These chemicals are commonly known as "feel good" chemicals and are what gives you energy after a workout. Stretching speeds up the recovery process and thus endorphin production occurs at a faster rate. As a result, you feel energized and ready to go sooner.

Pain minimization

Aching and tense muscles often lead to injury. Stretching after a workout reduces the risk of this by loosening them and minimizing the pain you may experience.

Better coordination

Stretching muscles after a workout has been shown to increase their functional mobility (Cross, 2018). One of the reasons this occurs is because your muscles are forced to relax together as you stretch and, therefore, you learn to work better in tandem. The result is that they synchronize better and your effective strength increases.

Mind-body connection

Stretching helps slow the body down gradually instead of abruptly stopping it after a workout. Stretching involves slow breathing and observing the muscles. This increases the connection your mind has with your body and you will become more aware of what is happening inside you.

The result is a greater sense of peace and awareness and a better overall mood. Now that you understand the benefits of stretching after training, let's take a look at the routine itself.

Your post workout routine

Follow this post-workout stretching routine step-by-step to maximize recovery. Hold these positions for 12 seconds to bring the muscles back to their original length. You can hold the poses for up to 20 seconds to increase flexibility.

Step # 1 Pectoral stretch

Stand a few feet from a pole or any vertical structure you can hold. Extend one hand backwards with the palm facing up and push the hand against the frame to stretch the upper chest. Repeat the movement with the other arm.

Step # 2 Stretching the lats

Stand in front of a wall a few meters away and raise one hand, palm fully open. Place it on the wall and gently press towards the wall. Repeat with the other arm.

Step # 3 Triceps and Back Stretch

Raise your arms and bend them at the elbow behind your head. Using the fingers of one hand, gently pull the elbow of the other arm inward until you feel a stretch in the triceps muscle. Repeat with the other arm.

Step # 4 Pectoral and rotator cuff stretch

Place your forearms on either side of a door and gently lean forward.

Step # 5 Calf stretch

Stand a few feet from a wall in front of it and lean forward to place your palms on the wall with one leg in front of the other. Repeat with the other leg.

Step # 6 Calf Stretch # 2

From the same position as in the previous exercise, place your back leg on your toe and gently bend your front knee towards the wall. Repeat with the other leg.

Step # 7 Quad Stretch

Stand on one leg and bend the other leg backward at the knee until you can grab your toes. Pull your toes to increase the stretch. Repeat with the other leg.

Step # 8 Stretch the hamstrings

Put one leg on a bench with the leg straight. Without bending the knee, lean forward as much as possible. Repeat with the other leg.

Step # 9 Hamstrings and Adductor Stretch

Rotate 90 degrees out from the previous position and the bed sideways towards the bench. Repeat with the other leg.

Step # 10 Stretching the adductors

Stand with your legs apart and lean forward as low as possible.

Step # 11 Adductors and calf stretch

Sit on your heels and squat as low as possible. Place your elbows on the inside of your knees and push your knees out.

Step # 12 Stretching the glutes

Sit on the floor and bend one leg 90 degrees at the knee. At the same time lift the other leg and place it outside the knee of the bent leg. Repeat with the other leg.

Step # 13 Cobra Stretch

Lie on the floor on your stomach and lift your chest off the floor with your palms firmly planted on the floor.

Step # 14 Cat Stretch

Get on all fours on your knees and palms. Make sure your head is in line between your palms. Now, bend your neck forward as you turn your upper back.

Breathing

One of the key things you can do to ensure better performance and to make sure you don't get injured is to breathe properly. Breathing is something that many beginners don't pay attention to and it's understandable. They focus on the correct form and weight they need to lift and forget that good breathing is part of the equation.

Breathing not only oxygenates the blood, but also helps firm the body against stress. If your body isn't firm at the right time during your workout, you could get injured. Knowing when to breathe isn't that complicated. Always remember to exhale during the exertion phase of an exercise.

For example, on the pushup, the effort phase is when you get off the ground. This means that you inhale as you descend and exhale as you push up. In a pull-up, the effort phase is when you pull yourself up and inhaling is when you lower yourself. Then inhale on the way down and exhale on the way up.

One of the other benefits of breathing properly is that as the blood becomes more oxygenated, it burns fat and carbohydrates more efficiently. In other words, not only does your body feed itself better, it also burns fat faster. Further weight loss is also achieved due to the fact that the body is better able to excrete excess water and toxins under such conditions.

So always remember to breathe correctly. At first, do the exercises slowly to get used to the rhythm of your breathing, and as time goes by, you will adapt.

EXERCISES

Workouts at home include bodyweight exercises, dumbbell exercises, and variations of the resistance band. You should have two different strength bands on hand before week 2 for home workouts. If you want to add more options to your workout, you will find a variety of dumbbells at most sporting goods stores. You may want to consider buying dumbbells of two different weights (see here for dumbbell weight guidelines). In general, you will use the lighter bands and weights for the smaller muscle groups, and you will use the heavier bands and weights for the larger muscles, such as the legs.

Gym workouts include dumbbells, bodyweight, gym machines, and a stability ball. Most gyms will have this equipment at your disposal.

Regardless of the equipment you use, correct form is key, so you target the right muscles and stay injury free. For each exercise, use controlled movements in both phases: lifting and lowering. Quick, jerky movements can cause injury. Slow down and focus on what you are doing and the muscles you are targeting. Remember, it shouldn't be easy, but that doesn't mean it can't be fun!

STATIC TRENDS: QUADRICEPS STRETCH

To properly stretch all quadriceps muscles, you will not only need to bend the knee, but stand straight enough to feel the stretch in the front hip of the standing leg.

Muscle groups: Quadriceps

INSTRUCTIONS

1. While standing on one straight leg, hold on to the countertop or back of a chair to help balance.

2. Bend the other knee back by grabbing the ankle with one hand.

3. It helps to bend the knee back as far as possible by gently pressing the foot towards the buttocks. If this causes stress on your knees, be very gentle.

4. Push your hips forward to engage them slightly to engage your hip flexors (the front of your hips where your legs meet your torso). Hold for 15-30 seconds (don't forget to breathe).

5. Return to standing position. Repeat with the opposite leg.

6. Repeat two or three times on both sides.

7. Safety tip: Be careful not to pull too hard if you experience knee pain. If so, press gently only until you feel a slight pull in the quadriceps.

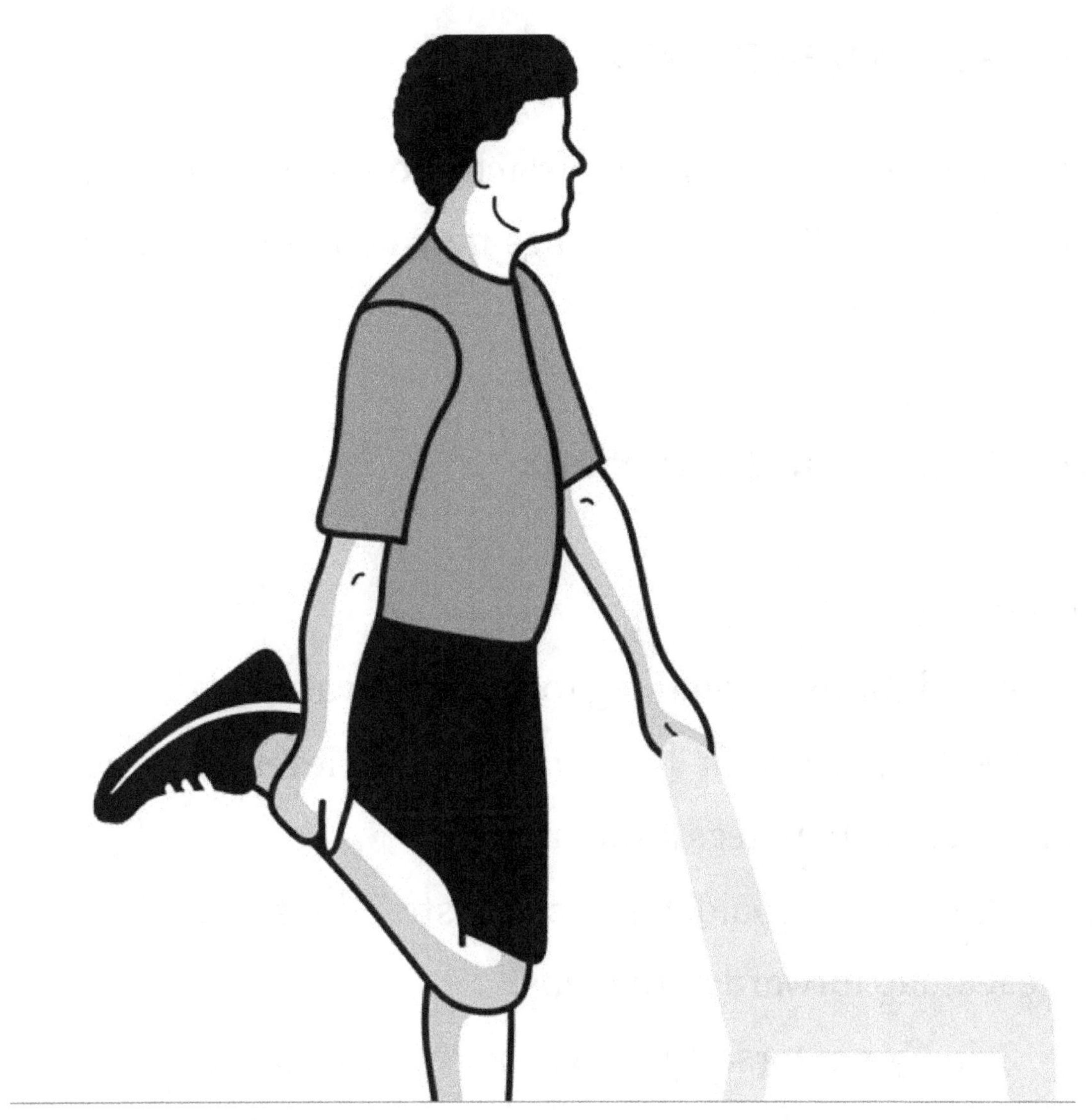

HAMSTRING STRETCH

It is especially important to stretch the hamstrings well before exercise. Tight hamstrings may be more prone to tension or tearing.

Muscle groups: Hamstrings

INSTRUCTIONS

1.   Avoid throwing your leg to a high elevation.

2.   Gently place your heel on a surface level with the chair, keeping both legs straight.

3.   The spine should be kept as straight as possible while leaning forward at the hips.

4.   Bring your torso towards the leg, without curving the spine. Hold the position for 15-30 seconds. (Don't forget to breathe.)

5.   Repeat with the opposite leg.

6.   Feel free to repeat two or three times.

Safety tip: Be careful not to curve your spine towards the extended leg.

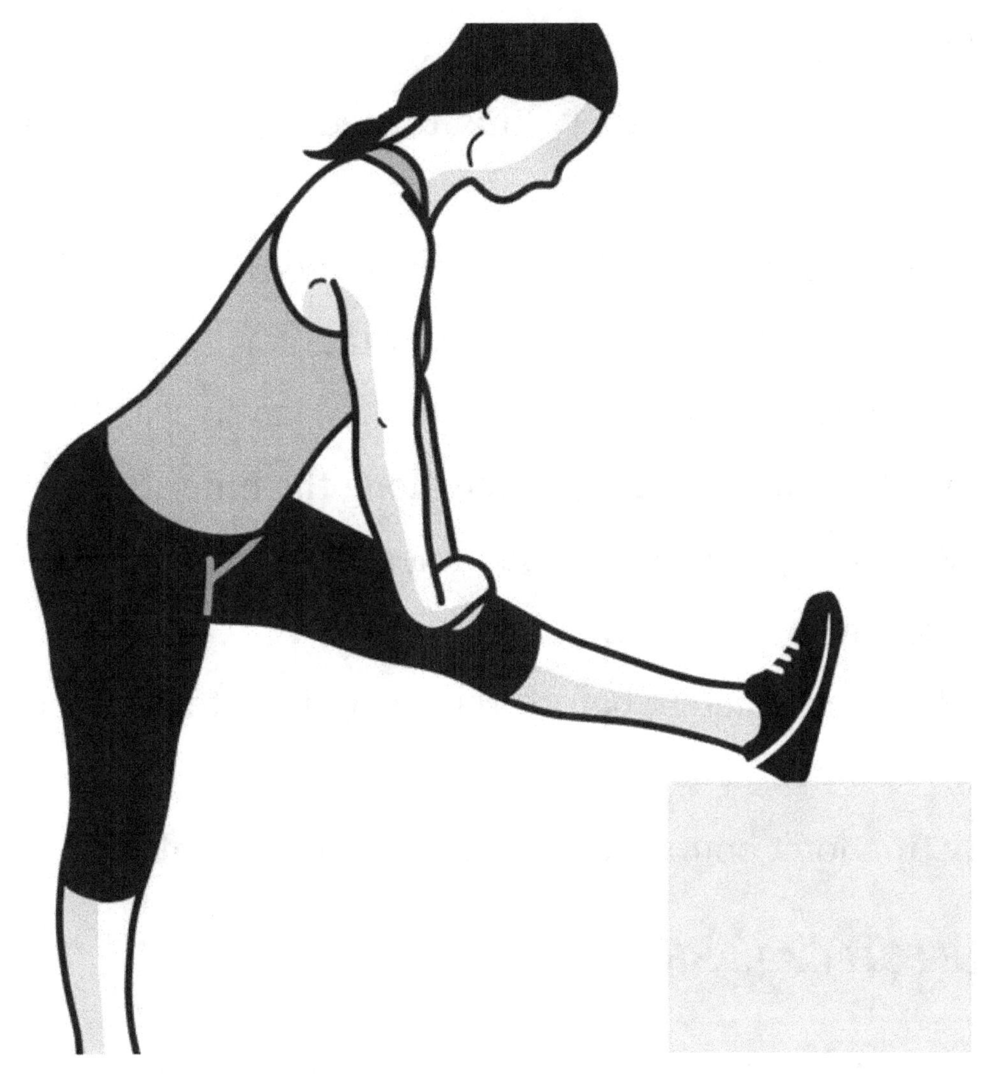

ELONGATION OF THE INNER THIGH

This stretch protects the hips by helping to maintain and improve the outward rotation of the hips.

Muscle groups: Groin adductors

INSTRUCTIONS

1.   Sit with feet together, hips turned out, knees bent, back straight, chin level.

2.   Bring your feet as close to your body as possible while allowing your knees to spread comfortably.

3.   Keeping your back straight, gently lean forward from your hips until you feel a slight stretch along the inner thigh.

4.   Rest your elbows on your knees to hold the position for 15-30 seconds. To breathe.

5.   Relax completely before repeating the steps two or three times.

Safety tip: don't bounce your legs. Just press gently and hold.

STRETCH CALFSKIN

These muscles play an important role in walking and running, and any level of tension can lead to pain and imbalance in other areas of the body. It is especially important to stretch your calf muscles if you wear high heels often or if you sit at a desk for long periods of time.

Muscle groups: Soleus Gastrocnemius

INSTRUCTIONS

1.   Start by standing two to three feet away from a wall, depending on your height.

2.   Place one foot in front of your body as you lean towards the wall.

3.   Place your hands against the wall at chest height. Keep your heels, hips and head in a straight line and your feet flat on the floor.

4.   Lean forward as you press your rear heel to the floor, until you feel a stretch in your calves. Hold the position for 15-30 seconds. (Don't forget to breathe.)

5.   To stretch the soleus, move away from the wall, standing more upright.

6.   Gently bend the back leg until you feel the stretch further down towards the heel. Hold the position for 15-30 seconds.

Safety tip: Avoid this stretch if you are experiencing Achilles tendon problems.

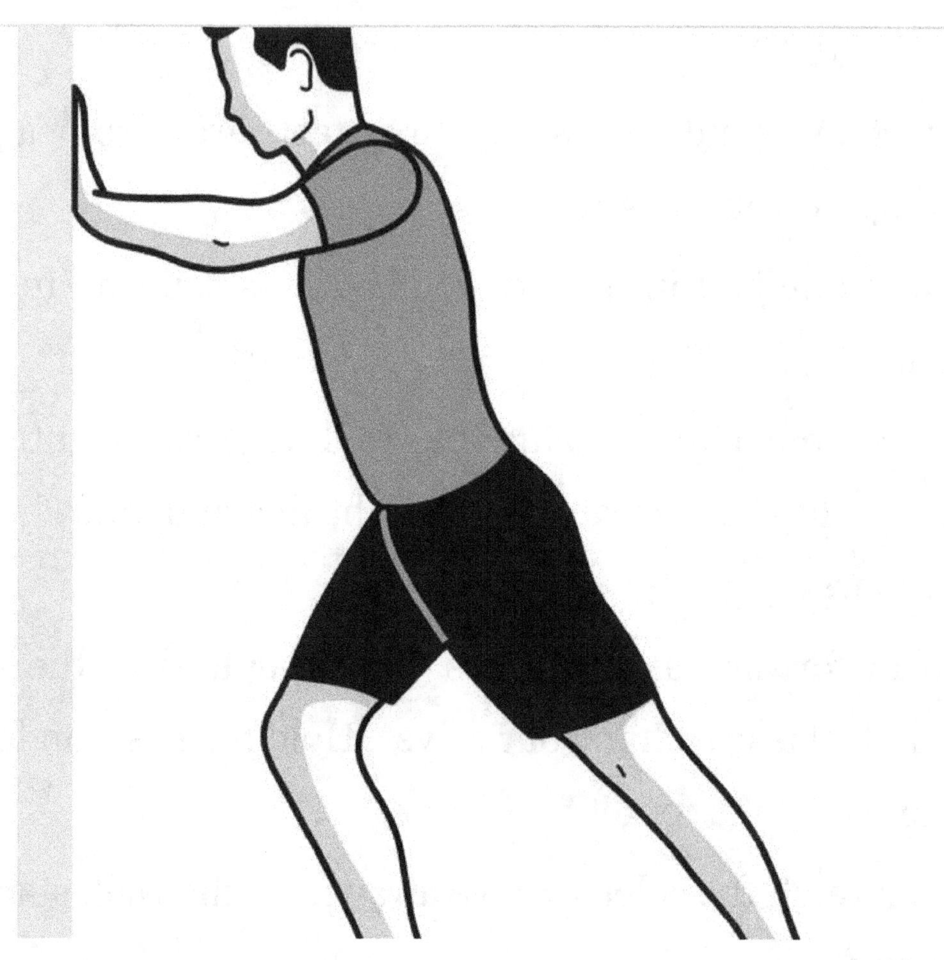

STATIC TRENDS: Latissimus Dorsi

INSTRUCTIONS

1.   Find a ledge that is approximately chest height, such as a fireplace mantle, or simply place your hands on a wall at the same height.

2.   Put your hands shoulder-width apart. Without moving your arms, slowly bend forward at your hips. Let the head fall towards the chest.

3.   Stop when you feel a stretch along the sides of your upper and middle back. (Don't forget to breathe.) Hold the position for 15-30 seconds, then relax.

4.   Repeat two or three times.

Safety tip: Avoid this stretch if you have shoulder pain.

ELONGATION OF THE BACK

The latissimus dorsi are the large, broad muscles located on each side of the upper and middle back.

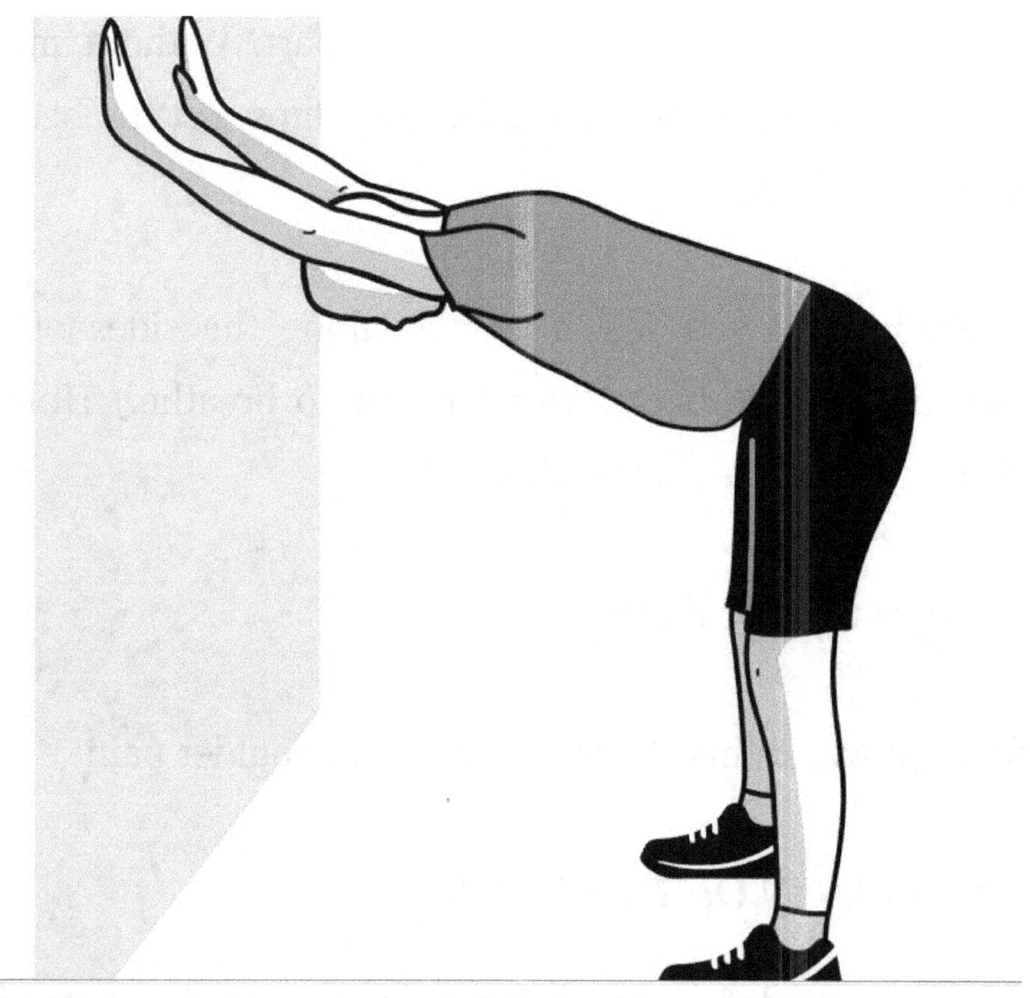

STATIC TRENDS: CHEST STRETCH

One of the most important muscle groups to stretch are the pectoral muscles, more commonly known as the chest muscles.

Muscle groups: Pectoral

Pectoralis minor anterior deltoid

INSTRUCTIONS

1.   Stand at right angles of two walls or in a door.

2.   Place your left arm 90 degrees on the door jamb or edge of the wall. Gently rotate your body away from that arm, away from the working side.

3.   You may need to move your feet slightly to point away from the working side. Additionally, you may need to rotate the non-functioning shoulder back slightly to feel the stretch. (You should feel the stretch in the front of the armpit on the working side.)

4.   Hold for 15-30 seconds on each side. (Don't forget to breathe.)

Safety tip: Be careful when turning your torso away from the point of contact.

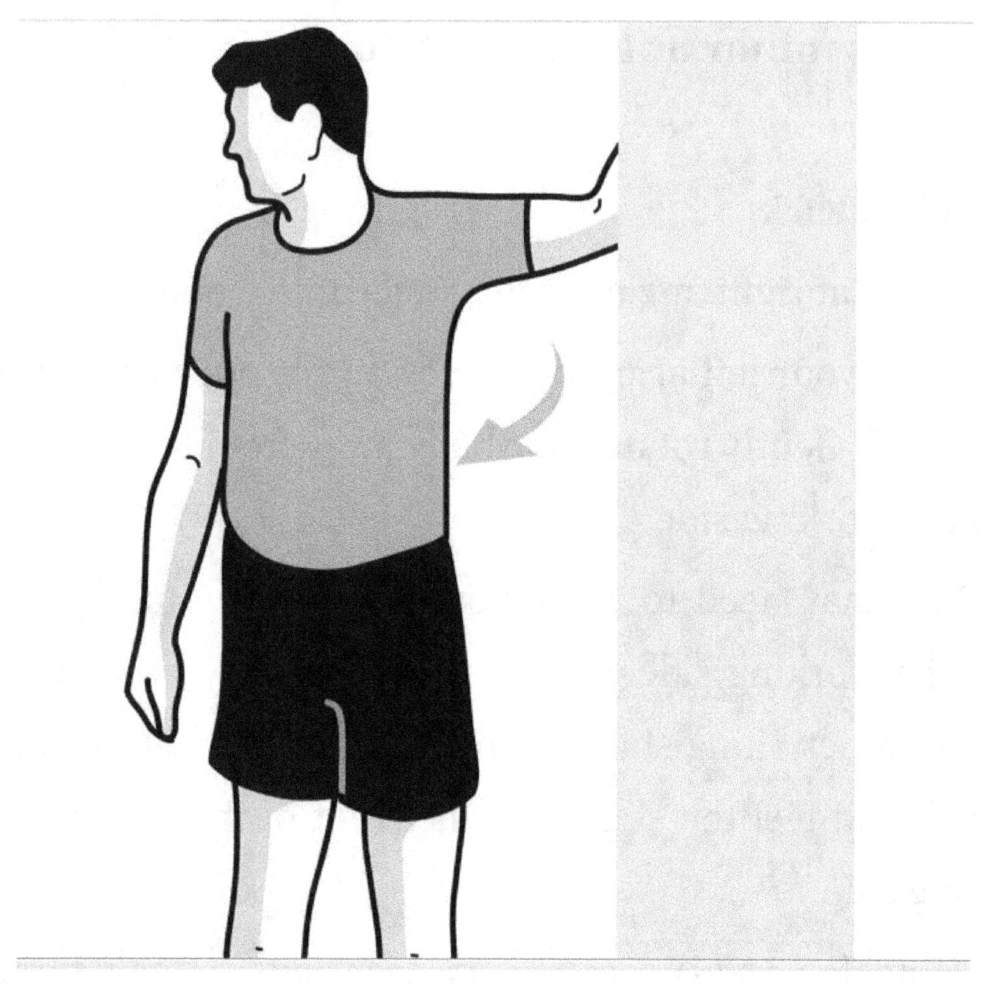

STATIC TRENDS: LOWER BACK STRETCH

Quadratus Lumborum

The quadratus lumborum is the deepest abdominal muscle and is found in the lower back, on either side of the lumbar spine.

INSTRUCTIONS

1. From a standing position, place one hand on your hip and raise the other arm above your head.

2. Bend to the side, extending the raised arm and reaching for the opposite side. (You can adjust where the stretch hits by lightly reaching the front of the body.)

3. Tuck your chin and look at the floor. Hold this position for 15 to 30 seconds. (Don't forget to breathe.)

4. Repeat on the other side.

5. To increase the stretch, hold one wrist with the opposite hand as you stretch or cross one leg in front of the other.

Safety tip: Be careful not to lean back. Stay neutral or lean slightly forward.

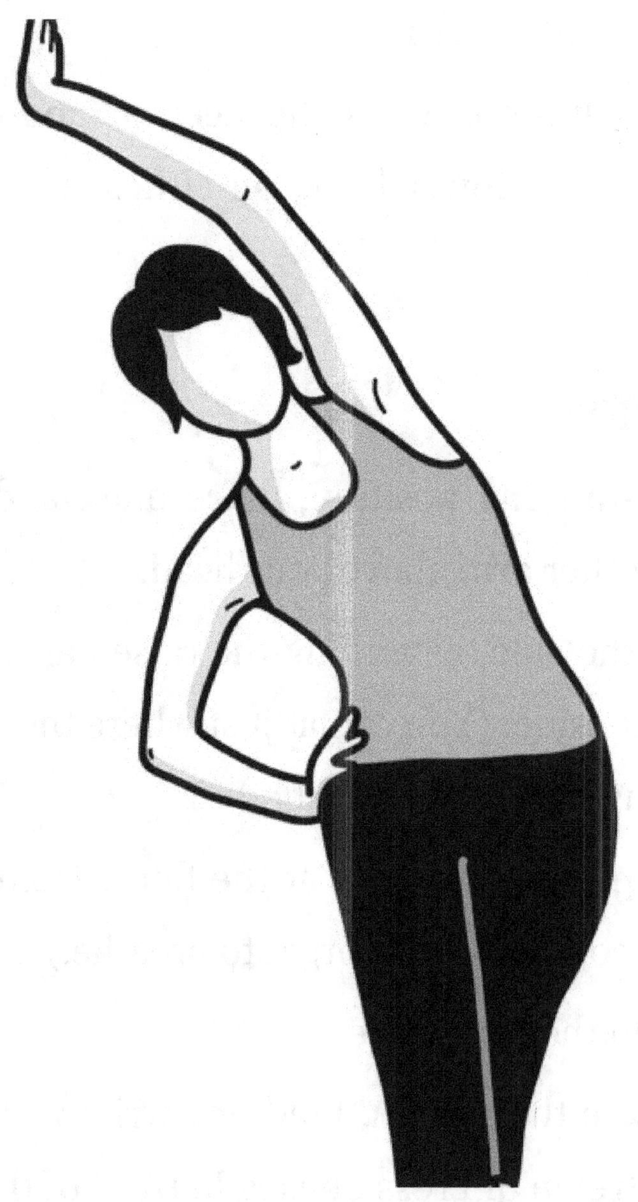

STATIC TRENDS: Piriformis

INSTRUCTIONS

1.   Lie on your back, bend both knees and bring your left ankle over your right thigh.

2.   Lift your right foot off the ground, bringing your leg to a 90 degree angle.

3.   Wrap your hands between your legs and slowly bring your right knee towards your chest.

4.   Keep your head and neck relaxed on the ground, holding the position for 15-30 seconds. (Don't forget to breathe.)

5.   Repeat on the other side.

6.   You can also do this stretch in a seated position by placing your ankle on the opposite knee and bending forward until you feel it stretch deep into the back of the hip.

Safety tip: If you are doing the seated version, be careful not to curve your spine forward. Keep your back straight as you lean forward.

DEEP HIP ELONGATION

If the piriformis pushes against the sciatic nerve (often caused by too much sitting), it can cause excruciating pain. muscle groups

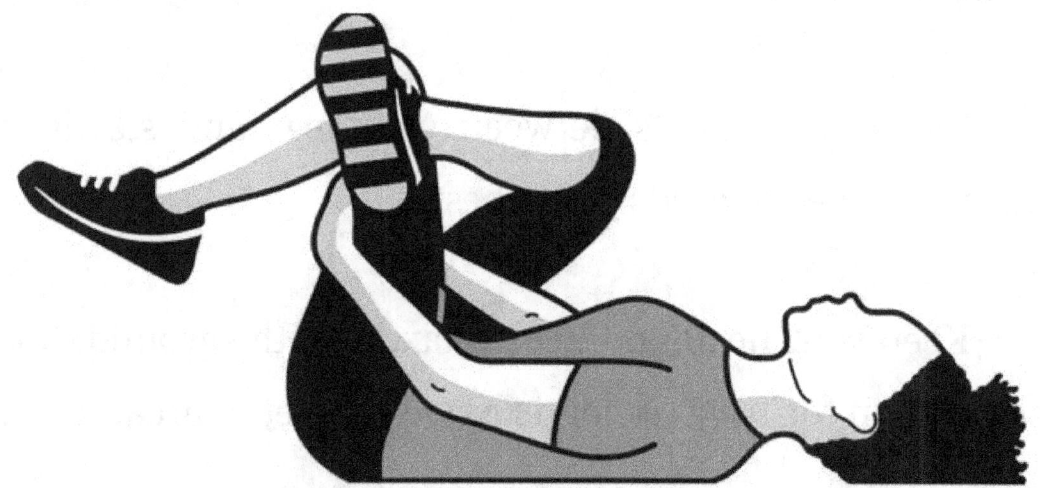

Static stretching program (take it easy)

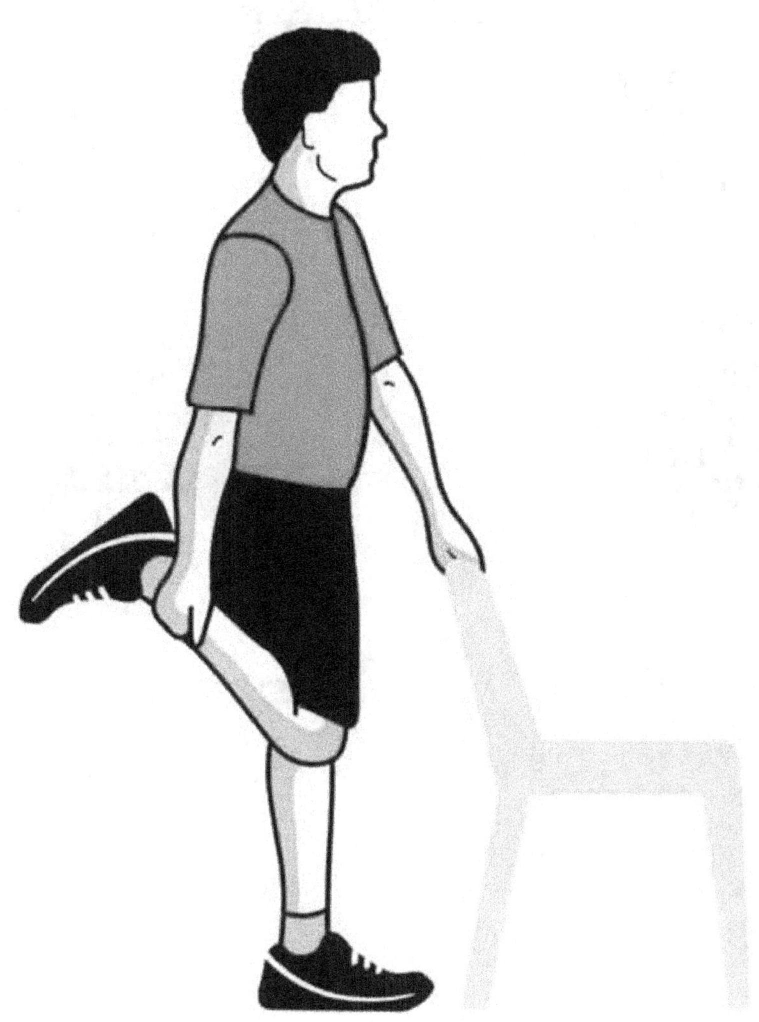

QUADRICEPS STRETCH

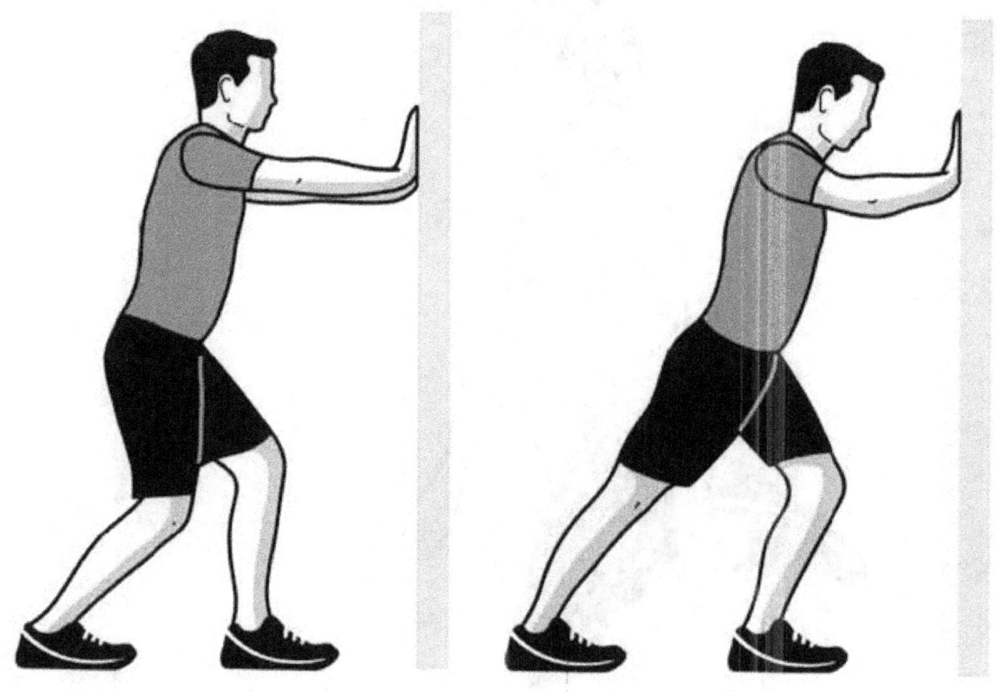

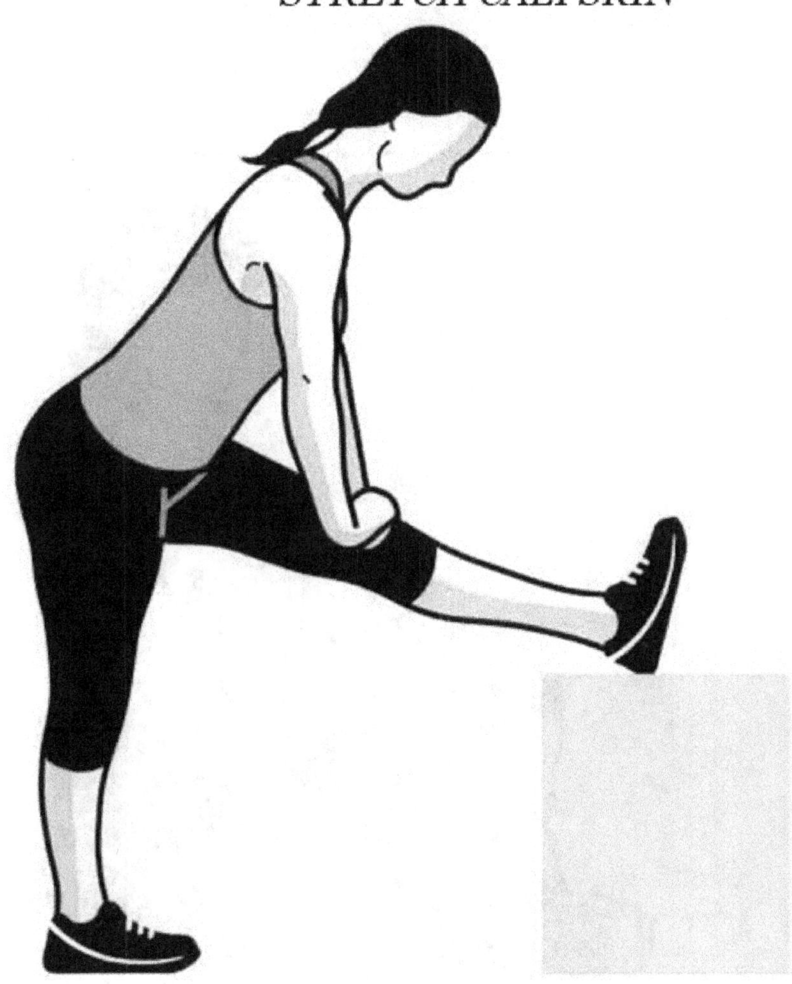

HAMSTRING STRETCH

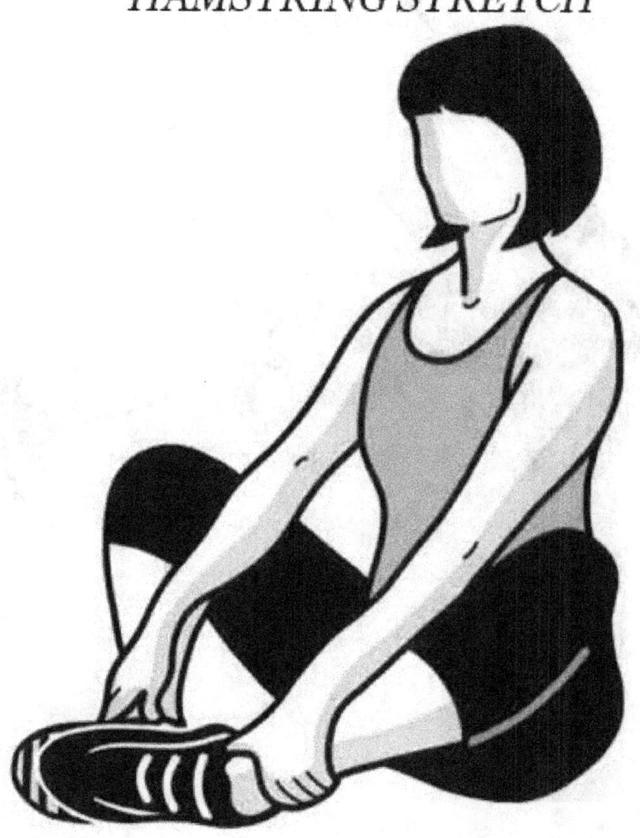

ELONGATION OF THE INNER THIGH

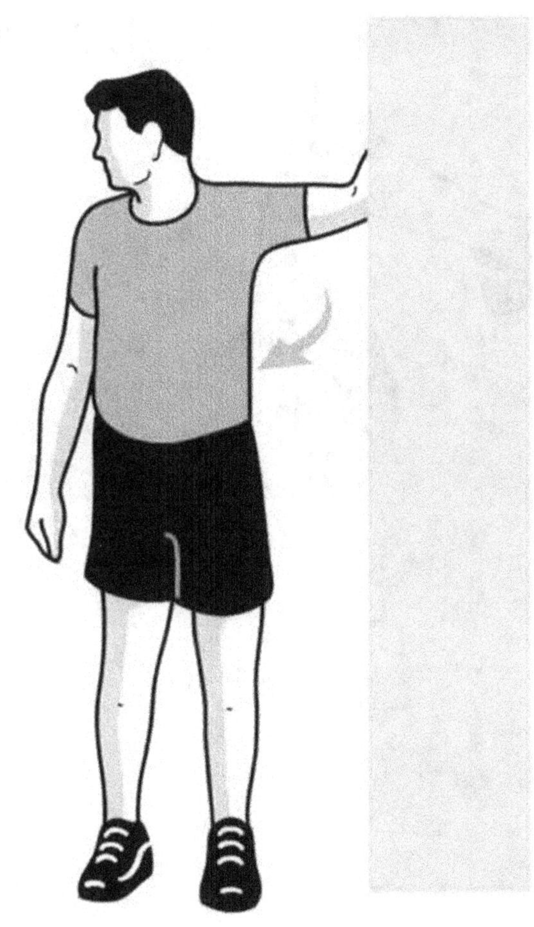

CHEST STRETCH

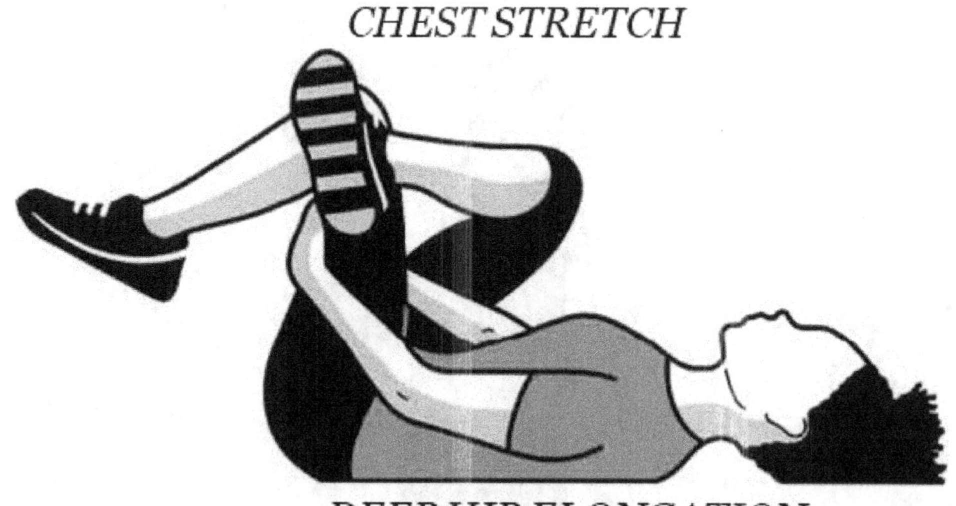

DEEP HIP ELONGATION

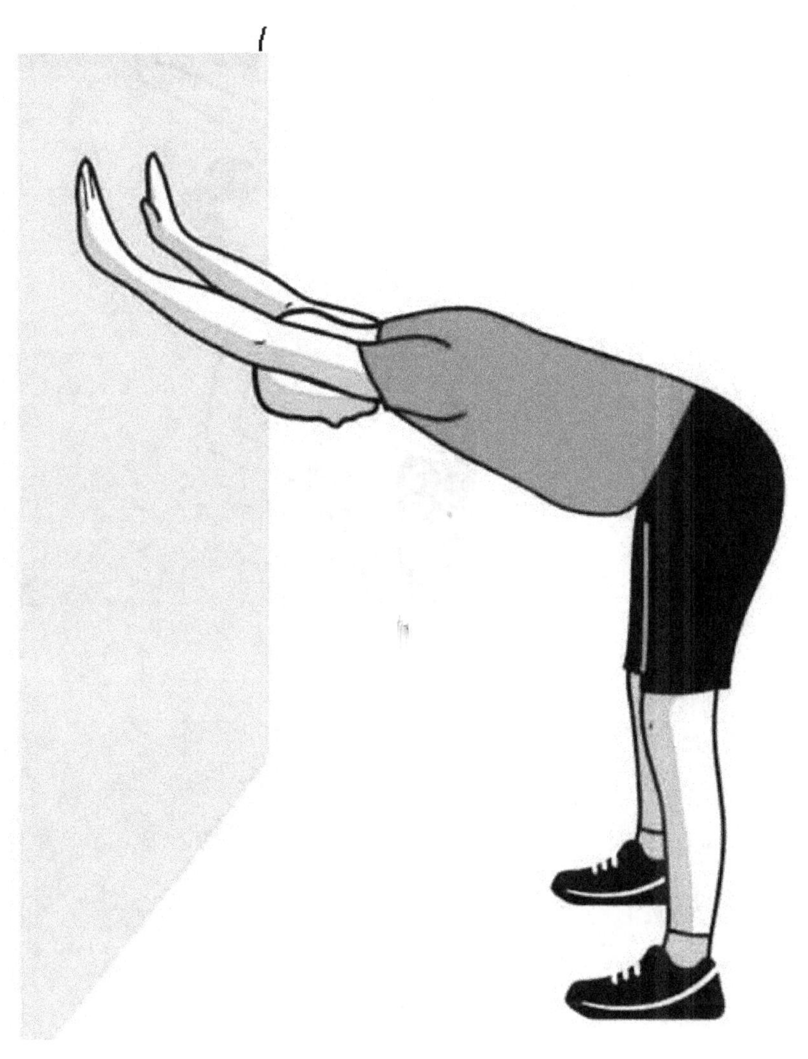

ELONGATION OF THE BACK

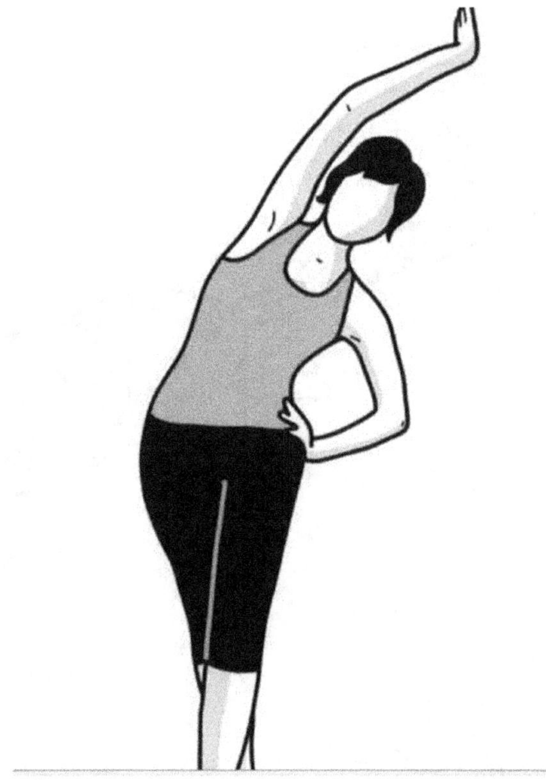

LOWER BACK STRETCH

Bodyweight exercises are a great way to start with strength training, although they have limitations due to the difficulty of adding resistance. There are ways, however, to modify bodyweight exercises over time to make them more difficult. For example, you can add time to the plank, add repetitions to all exercises and slow down the movements.

FOREARM PLANK

The plank is an essential exercise for building core strength for any level. The goal is to hold the position for a set amount of time, or as long as possible without dropping or lifting your hips.

Muscle groups: Rectus abdominis

Spinal erectors

Transverse abdominals

INSTRUCTIONS

1.   Draw a straight line from the shoulders to the heels, keeping the neck neutral looking down.

2.   Keep your elbows under your shoulders. Stay relaxed and breathe.

3.   Hold the position for as long as possible (up to 60 seconds).

Safety tip: Press and hold your navel to prevent your back from arching or bending.

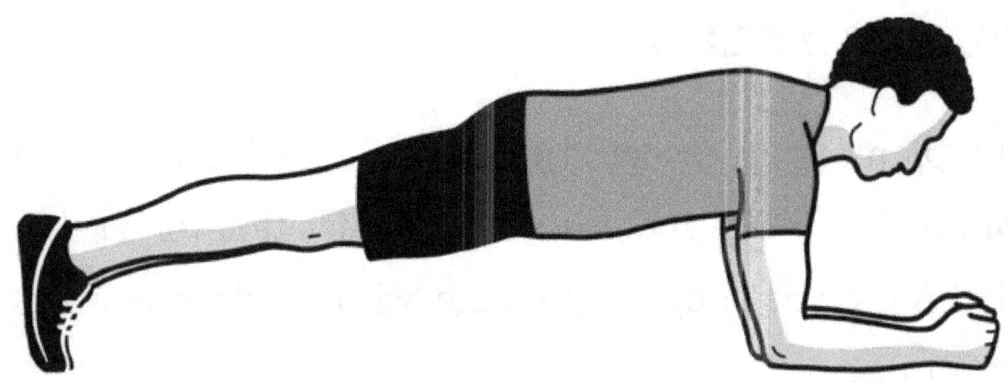

PARTIAL CRUNCH

Partial crunches are superior to sit-ups because they use the part of a sit-up where the muscles are fully engaged.

Muscle groups: Rectus abdominis

(With focus on the bottom)

INSTRUCTIONS

1.   Lie on your back with your knees bent and feet flat on the floor.

2.   Put your hands behind your head. It is better not to interlace your fingers. You can also cross your arms across your chest if that's more comfortable.

3.   Gently pull your abs inward.

4.   Bend up and forward so that your head, neck, and shoulders lift off the floor.

5.   Aim for two sets of 10 to 15 reps.

6.   For more of a challenge, keep your legs 90 degrees as you perform the exercise.

Safety tip: Make sure you don't pull your neck as you lean up.

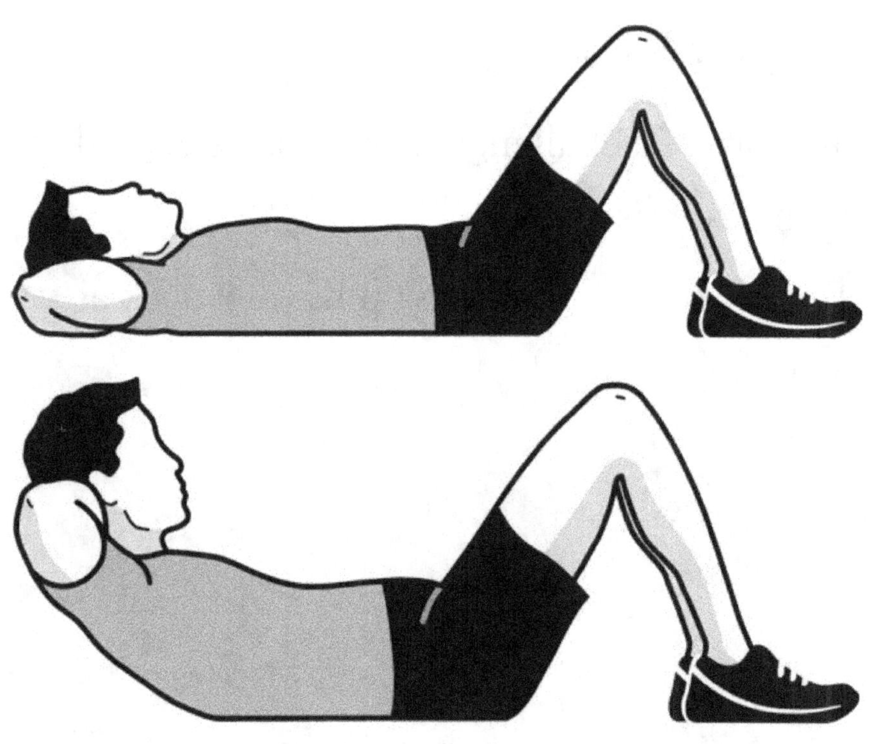

REVERSE CRUNCH

The reverse crunch is a popular exercise that targets the abs, especially the lower body.

Muscle groups: Rectus abdominis

(With focus on the bottom)

INSTRUCTIONS

1.   Lie on your back with your hands under your hips.

2.   Bend your knees and lift them towards your head, keeping your knees bent at 90 degrees.

3.   Draw them slightly upwards at the end of the movement. Be careful not to use momentum to swing your legs over your head. Focus on the abdominal muscles which act like an accordion to "bend" the bent legs at the torso.

4.   For a more advanced version, try lifting your hips off the floor while your legs are at maximum motion. If you can't do this, with constant effort, as your core strengthens, you may find that you can lift your hips off the floor.

5.   Lower your feet to just above the floor, without fully extending your legs, to complete one rep. Repeat until the desired number of repetitions.

Safety tip: Do not allow your legs to fully extend when lowering. This is too hard for the lower back.

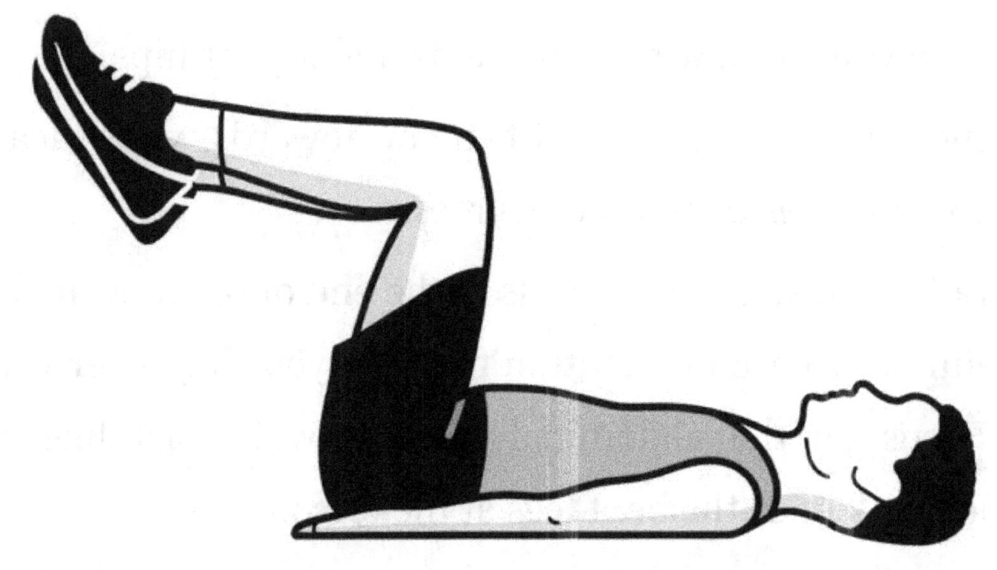

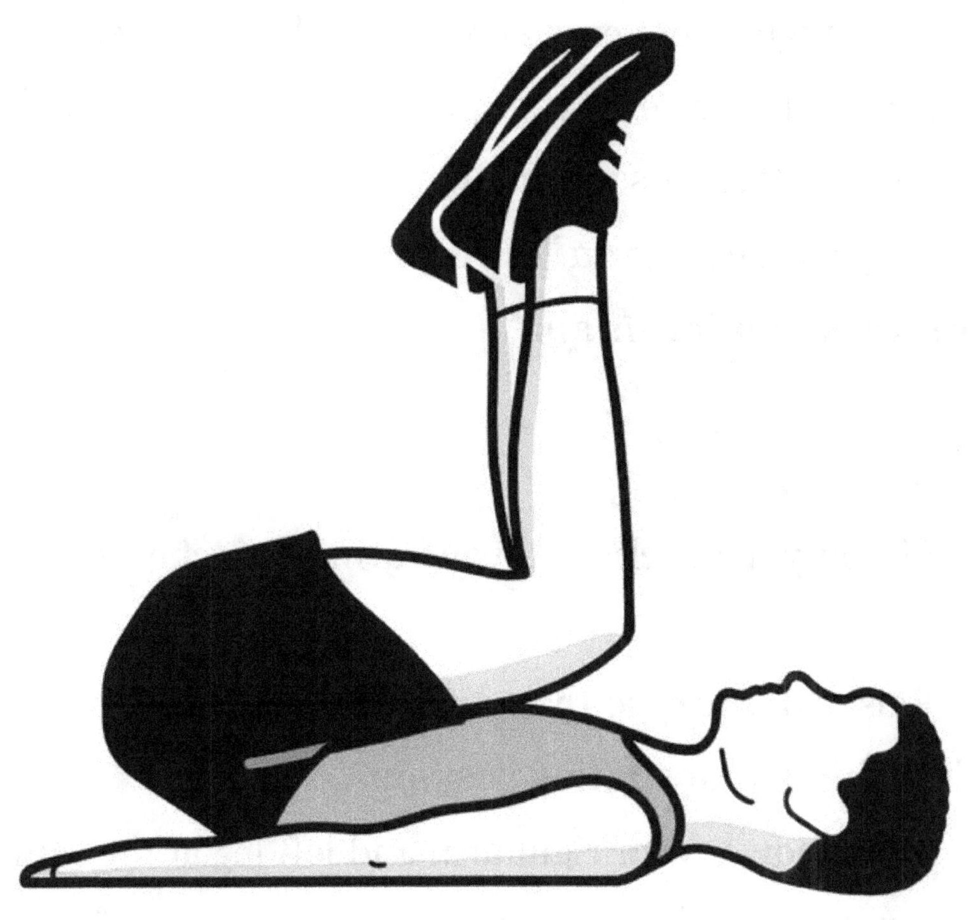

BUG DEAD

Dead bug might seem easy enough for the first two reps, but if you keep your core engaged, pressing your lower back to the floor will feel fatigue soon enough.

Muscle groups: Spinal erectors

Transverse abdominals

INSTRUCTIONS

1.   Lie on your back with your arms stretched towards the ceiling.

2.   Raise your legs so that your knees are bent at 90 degree angles. This is your starting position.

3.   Slowly lower your right arm and left leg at the same time, until your arm and leg are just above the floor. The arm and leg should be straight and fully extended.

4.   Then slowly return to the starting position, keeping the arm extended and bending the leg back 90 degrees. Repeat with opposite limbs.

5.   Use slow controlled movements when lowering and returning to the starting position. Make sure your back is flat against the floor during the movement.

6.   Aim for 10 reps on each side. Work up to two rounds of this exercise.

7.   For a more advanced version of the dead bug, keep your shoulders off the floor during the movement and be careful to keep the knee bent 90 degrees (the thigh of the leg not extended should be perpendicular to the floor).

Safety tip: Always keep the floor pressed against the floor.

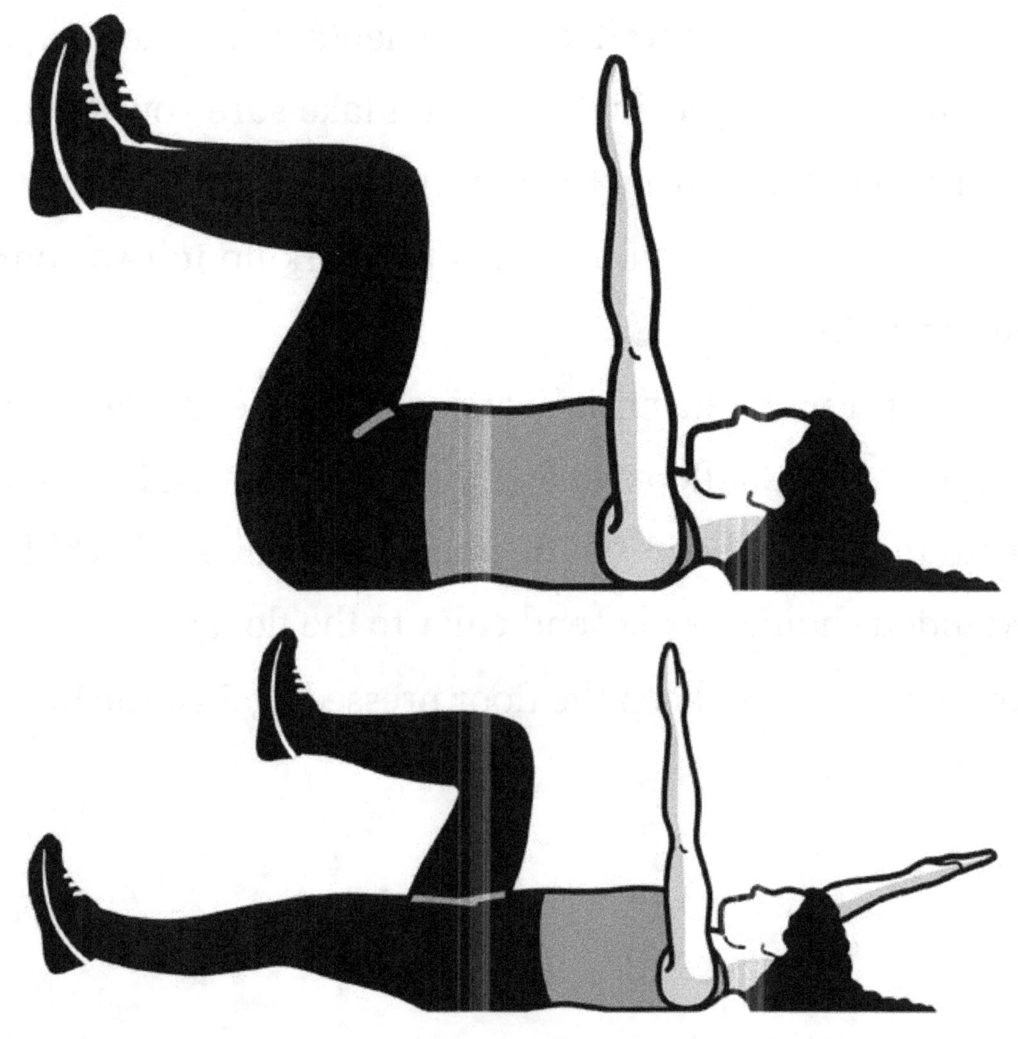

SIDE PLANK

This exercise targets a set of muscles that act as stabilizers.

Muscle groups: External obliques

Internal obliques

Transverse abdominal square of the loins

INSTRUCTIONS

1.	Lie on your side with your forearm flat on the floor, your lower elbow aligned directly under your shoulder, and both legs extend in a long line or bend 90 degrees for easier modification. Your upper hand can be on the hip side (easier) or reach the ceiling (more challenging).

2.	If the legs are extended, the feet can be staggered for greater stability or stacked for greater challenge.

3.	For an intermediate version, keep the lower leg bent but extend the upper leg out, actively engaging the inner thigh as you push the upper leg into the floor.

4.	Engage your core and lift your hips off the floor, forming a straight line from head to toe or head to knees for modification. Keep your hips pressed up. You should feel it mostly on the side closest to the floor.

5.	Hold the position for 15-30 seconds and increase to 60 seconds over time.

Safety tip: If you experience shoulder pain, it may be best to avoid it until the shoulder heals.

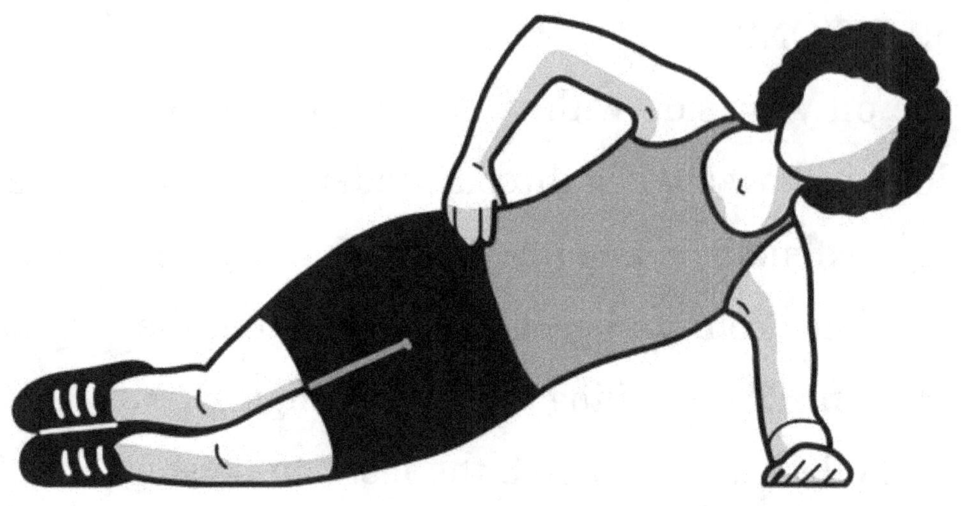

PUSH-UP (WITH VARIATIONS)

Knee push-ups (easier)

The more our body is parallel to the floor, the more challenging the movement.

Therefore, a chair push-up is more challenging than a table-height push-up. A push-up from the knees is easier than one from the toes.

Muscle groups: Pectoralis major quadriceps

Pectoralis minor anterior deltoid

INSTRUCTIONS

1. Start with the high board with stacked shoulders, elbows and wrists and a long spine.

2. Come on your knees. Your body should be in a straight line from the knees to the head.

3. Bend your elbows and lower your chest to the ground.

4. Push your palms to straighten your arms.

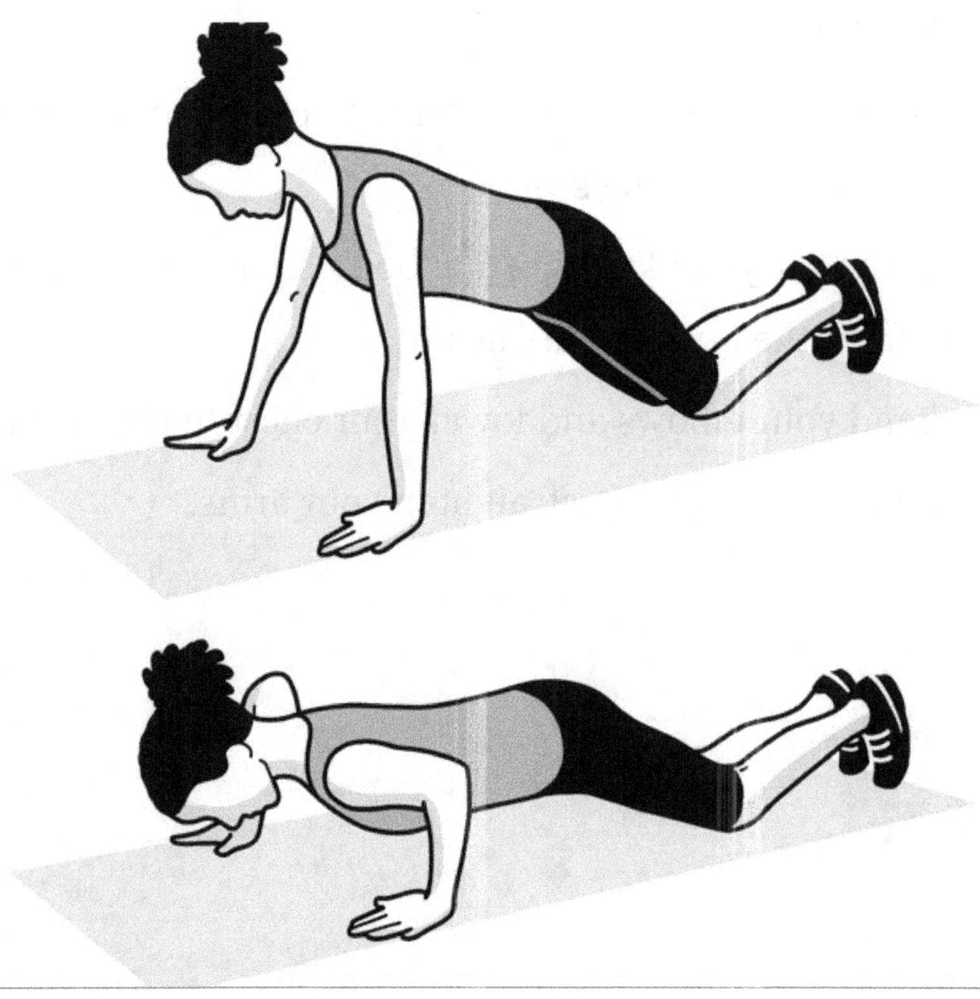

Table / Chair Push-Ups (Medium Challenge)

You can adjust the degree of challenge by varying the degree of your body. At home, some useful items to use are a table or chair. Make sure the items you are using are stable. You don't want them to move from under you. Keep your body in a straight line as you lower yourself and push back.

INSTRUCTIONS

1. Place an object, such as a chair, with its back against a wall.

2. Grab both sides of the chair seat and move your feet back until you are aligned from the tip of your head to your feet.

3. Engage your core by pulling inward on your navel.

4. Lower your chest towards the chair as comfortably as possible, while maintaining your shape. Avoid bending your elbow outward.

5. Push back while maintaining body alignment. Return to the starting position and repeat the desired repetitions.

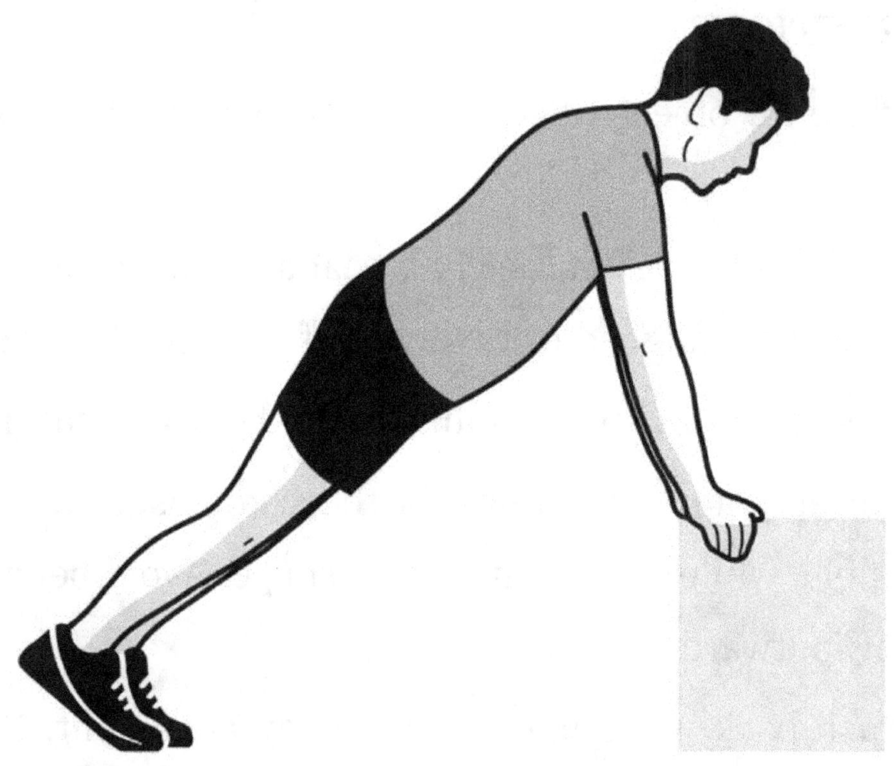

Toe push-ups with short stop (more challenging)

Fully extending your legs increases the difficulty of this move by adding more body weight.

INSTRUCTIONS

1. Start with your chest and stomach flat on the floor. Your legs should be straight behind you with your toes hidden. The palms of the hands should be level with the chest with the arms bent at a 45 degree angle.

2. Exhale as you push from your hands and heels, lifting your entire body off the floor.

3. Pause for a second in the straight-arm plank position, keeping your core engaged.

4. Inhale as you slowly lower yourself to the starting position.

Safety tip: Make sure the object you are using to lift yourself is stable and does not move from under you.

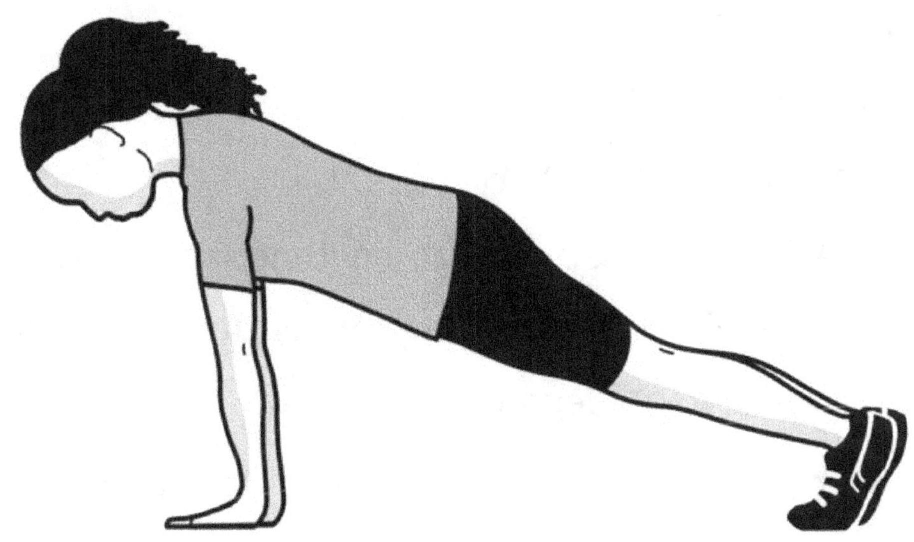

TRICEPS DIP (WITH VARIATIONS)

The triceps dip is a great exercise for anyone looking to strengthen the back of their upper arms, not just for aesthetic reasons but for added strength for any type of pushing movement.

Muscle groups: Anterior deltoid

Pectoral

Pectoralis minor triceps

Bent legs (easier)

INSTRUCTIONS

1. Sit on the edge of a chair or bench and grasp the edge with your hands.

2. Place your heels on the edge of the other chair and stand upright using your triceps.

3. Slide forward just enough so that your butt leaves the edge of the chair, then lower yourself until your elbows are bent as close to 90 degrees as possible.

4. Push back until your arms are straight, without using your legs to help push.

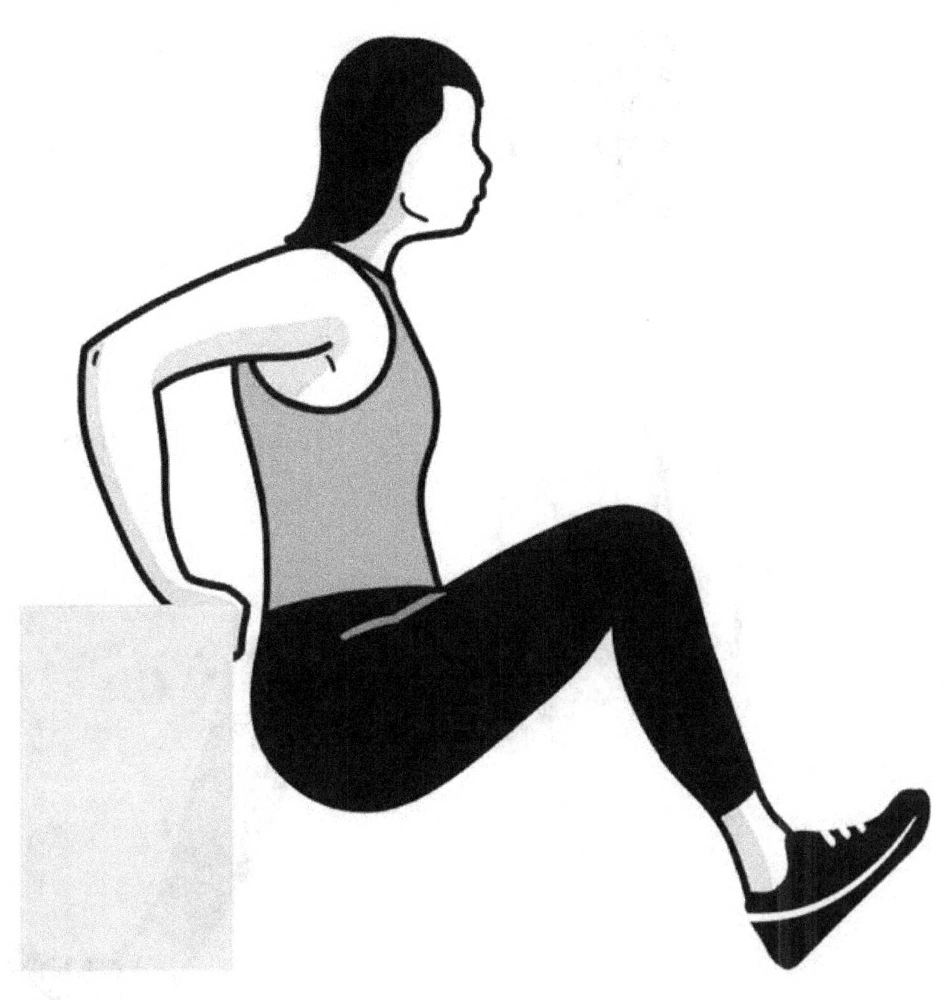

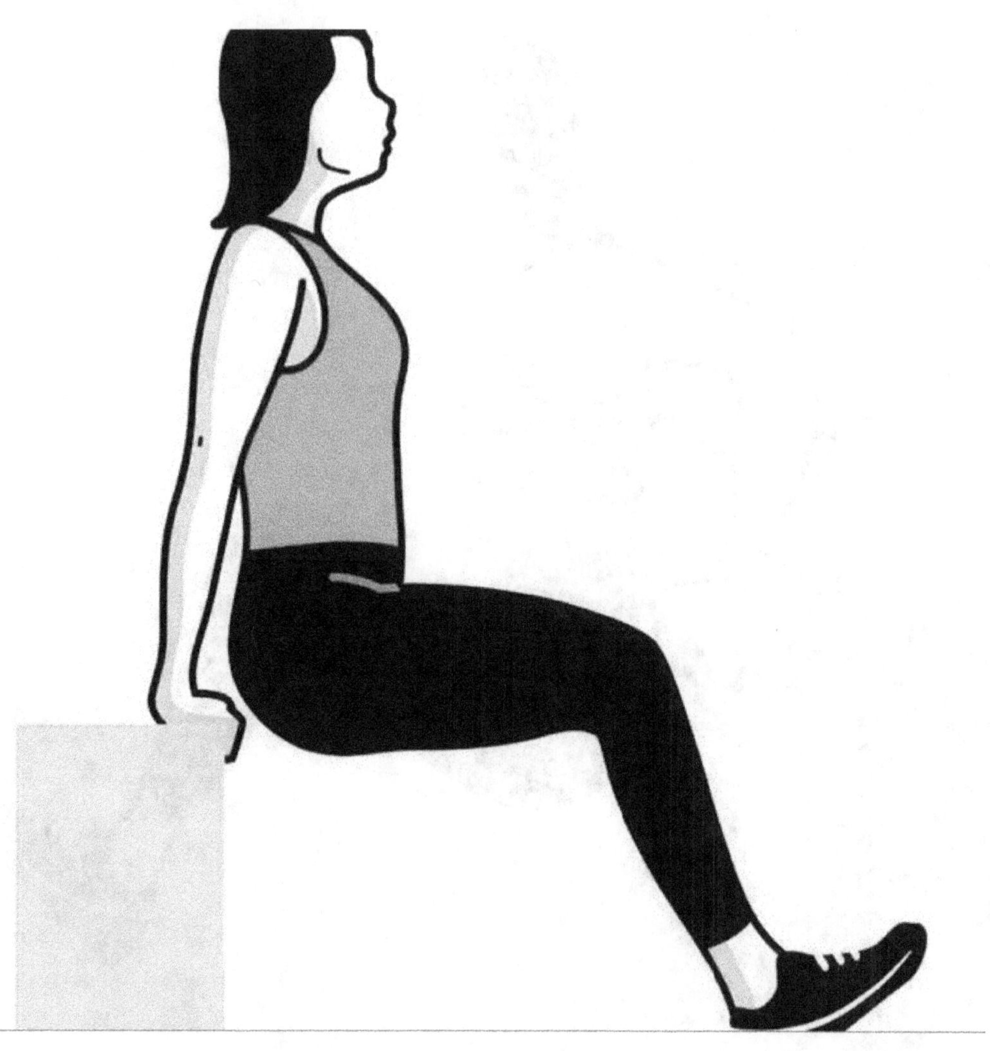

Straight leg (more demanding)

INSTRUCTIONS

1. Grab the front edge of an object at the height of the chair near your thighs.

2. Walk with your feet forward until your hips are slightly bent, with your legs straight and your arms outstretched.

3. Bend your elbows about 90 degrees and lower your hips towards the floor.

4. Push back to the starting position. Be careful not to lock your elbows too long, as it serves as a rest.

Safety tip: Lower yourself slowly so that you only go as far as your shoulders comfortably allow.

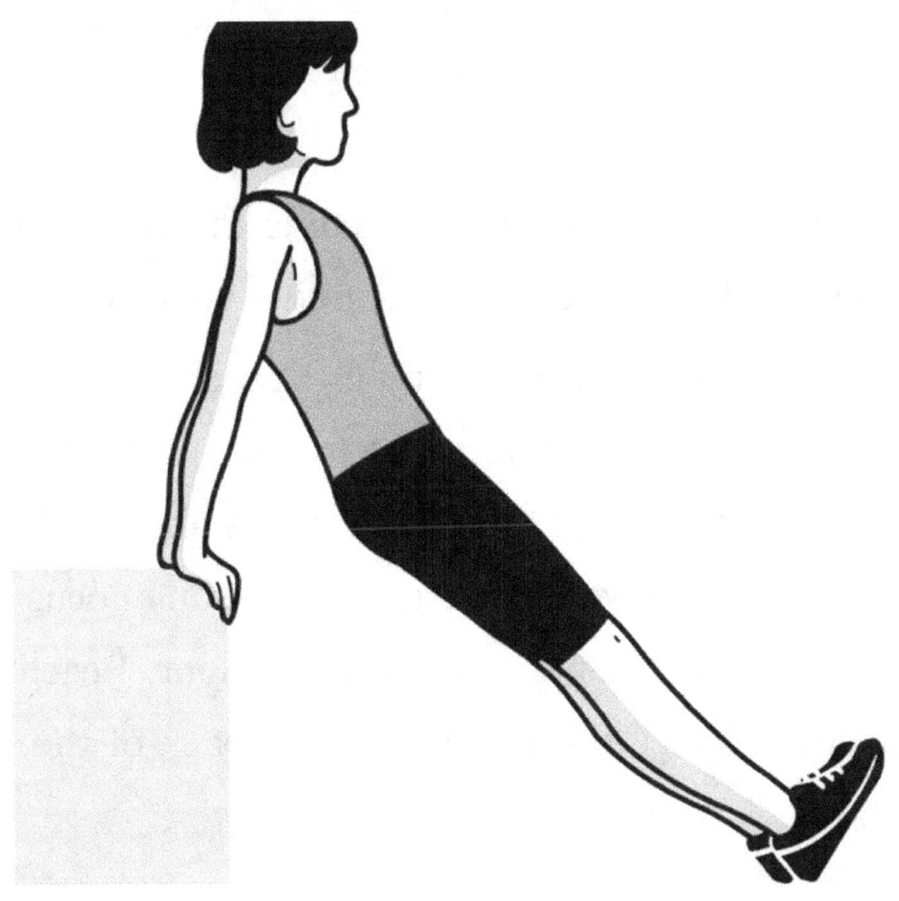

DOG BIRD

The bird dog engages the core and back muscles simultaneously. It is considered safe exercise when recovering from a back injury.

Muscle groups: Spinal erectors

Abs (to a lesser extent)

Buttocks (to a lesser extent)

Hamstrings (to a lesser extent)

INSTRUCTIONS

1. Start on all fours with your hands directly under your shoulders and your knees directly under your hips.

2. Bring your abs into your spine. Keeping your back and pelvis still and stable, stretch your right arm forward and your left leg back. Don't allow your pelvis to swing from side to side as you move your leg behind you. Focus on not letting your rib cage bend towards the floor. Reach for the left heel to engage the muscles in the back of the leg and glutes.

3. Return to the starting position, placing your hand and knee on the floor. Repeat on the other side to complete one rep.

4. Work up to 10-12 repetitions on each side.

Tip: Try to keep your hips perpendicular to the floor as you alternate limb extensions.

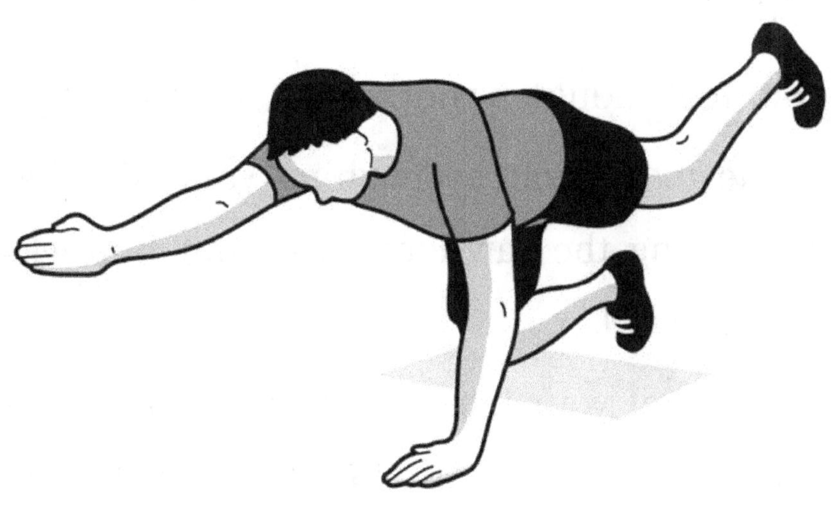

BODYWEIGHT SQUAT OR FREESTANDING SQUAT CHAIR

The squat is a fundamental movement that strengthens the lower body. It is important for beginners to learn the correct form before moving on to squats with weights (dumbbells, barbell).

Muscle groups: Buttocks

Quadriceps

INSTRUCTIONS

1. Put your feet shoulder-width apart, toes slightly out.

2. Begin the movement by pushing your hips back. (As if you were closing the car door with your buttocks because your hands are full.)

3. Slowly bend at your knees, continuing to push your hips back until your thighs are as close to parallel to the floor as possible.

4. At the end of the movement, stop for a second or two and push hard back to the starting position. Keep your chin parallel to the floor and keep your back straight.

5. Repeat until the desired number of repetitions.

Tip: If you find independent squats too difficult at first, use the chair to rest for a second before pushing back. Switch to the independent version as soon as you can comfortably.

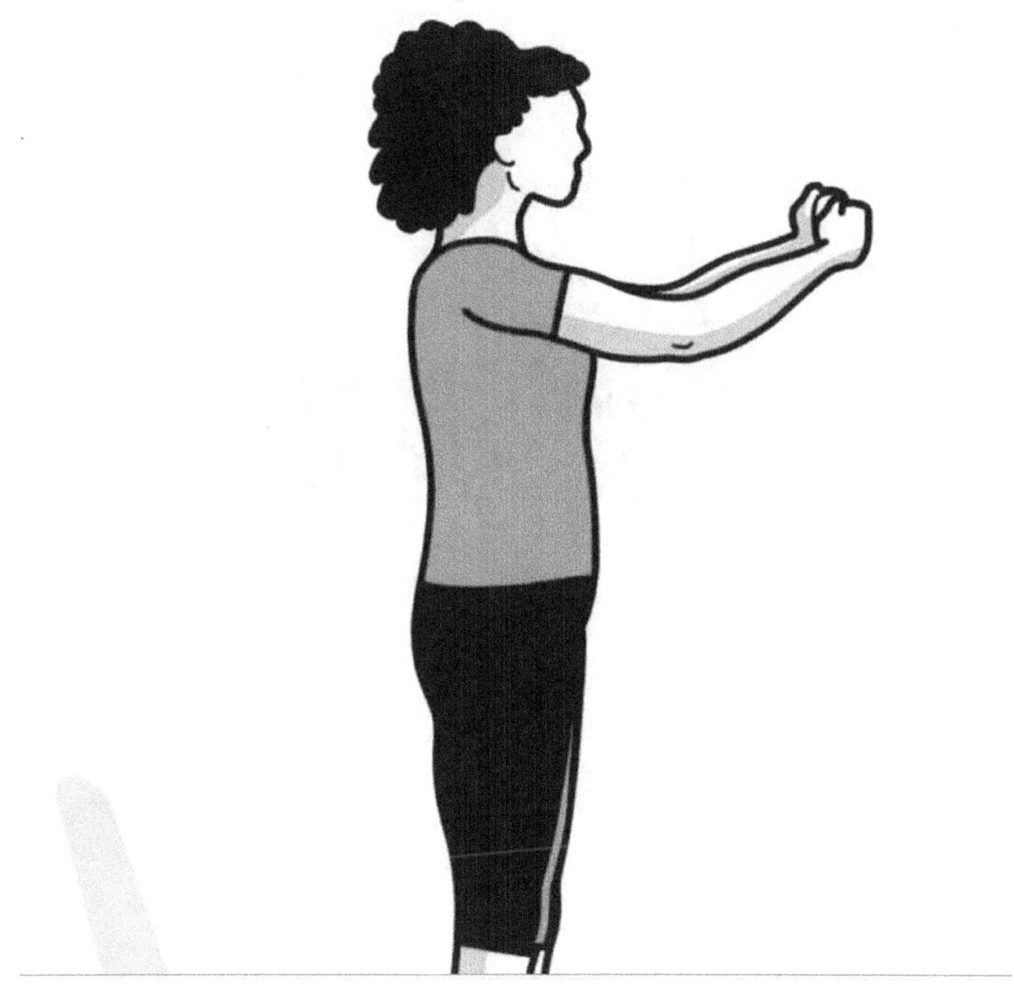

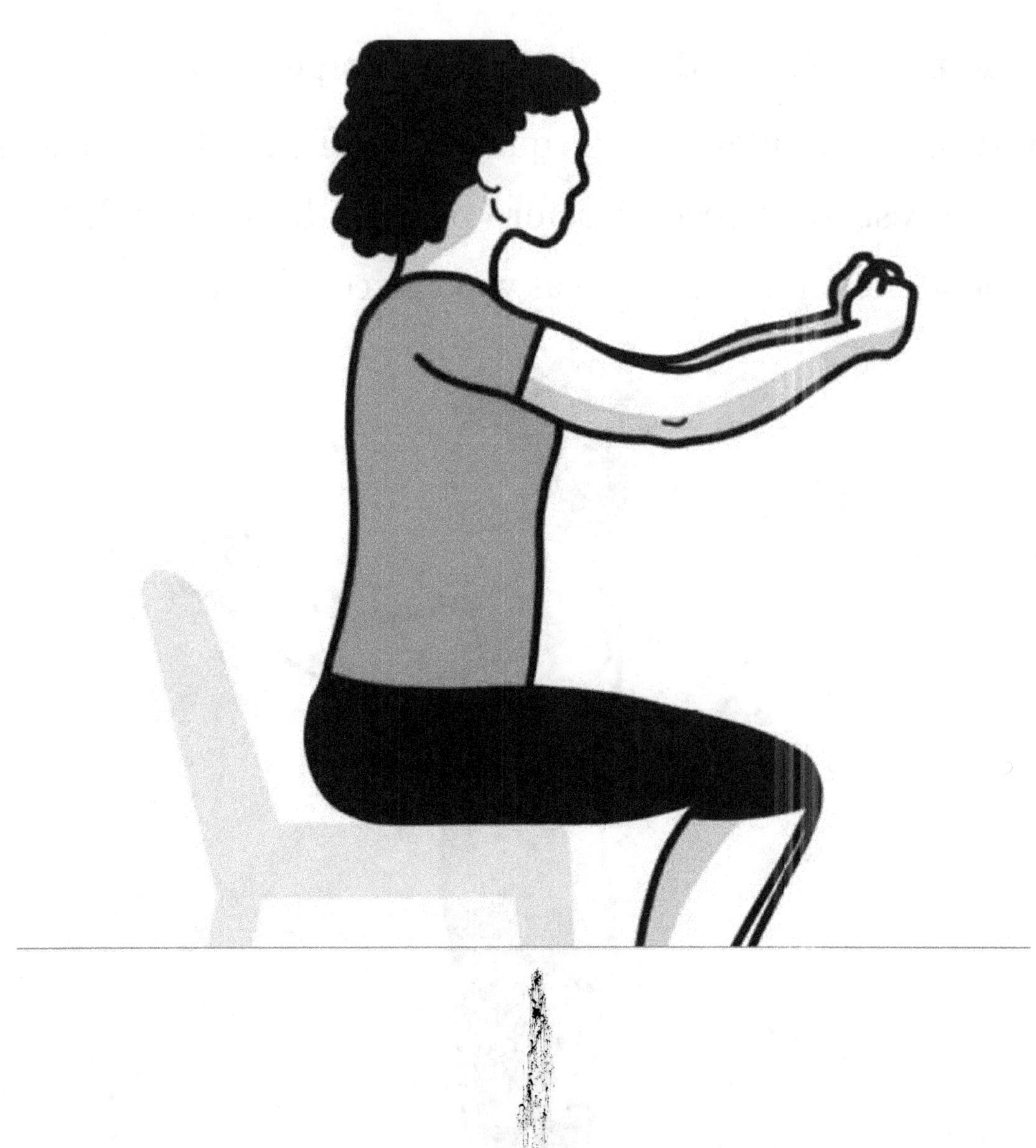

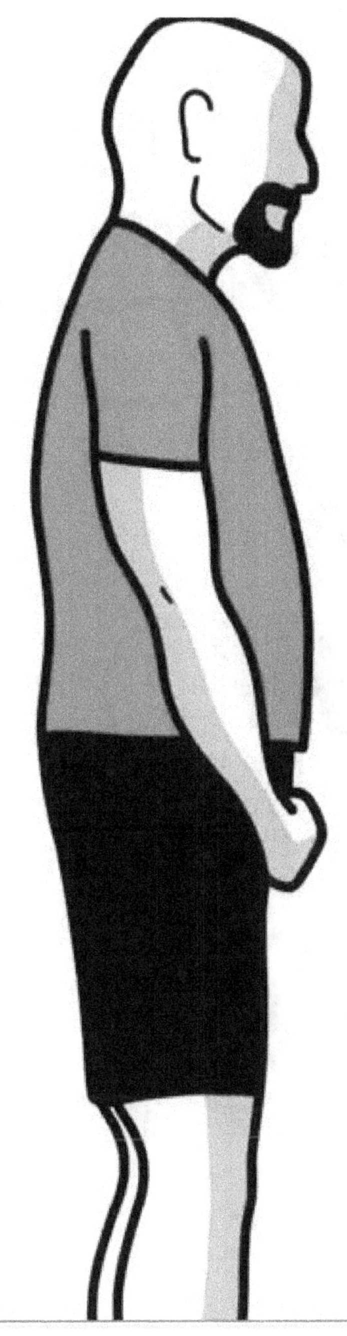

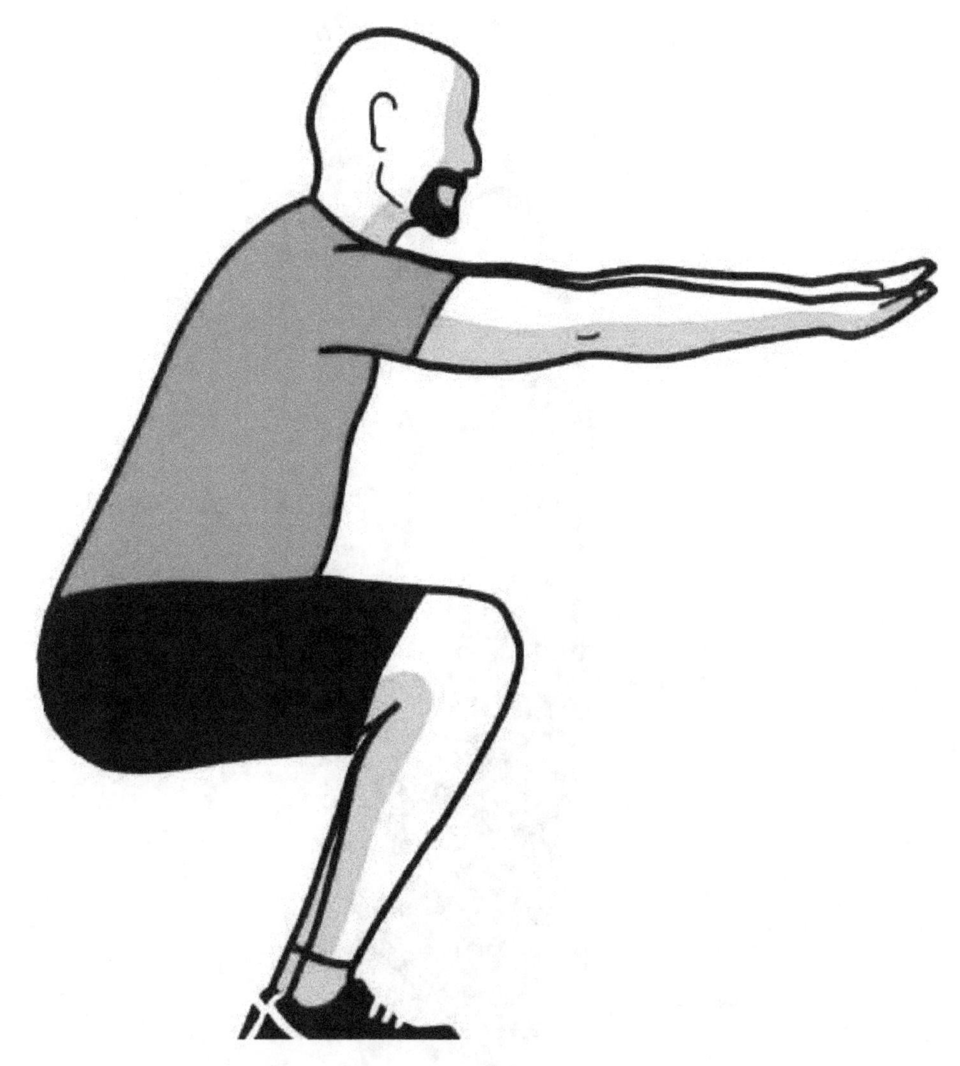

SQUAT SINGLE LEG WITH CHAIR OR BENCH (ADVANCED)

The single leg squat is an advanced alternative to basic bodyweight or chair squat, which requires no equipment. The bench or chair will serve as a resting place before pushing back. But don't sit for too long.

Muscle groups: Buttocks

Quadriceps

INSTRUCTIONS

1. Stand in front of a bench or chair and lift one leg slightly in front of you. The lower the rest point, the harder it will be.

2. Push your hips back and squat on the bench.

3. Try to barely touch the ground before standing upright. Your free foot will extend more towards the floor when you stand up, but will naturally come forward as you lower yourself.

4. Push your heel to the floor as you return to a standing position. Avoid moving your arms to get up.

Safety tip: Avoid this movement if you are experiencing SI joint problems.

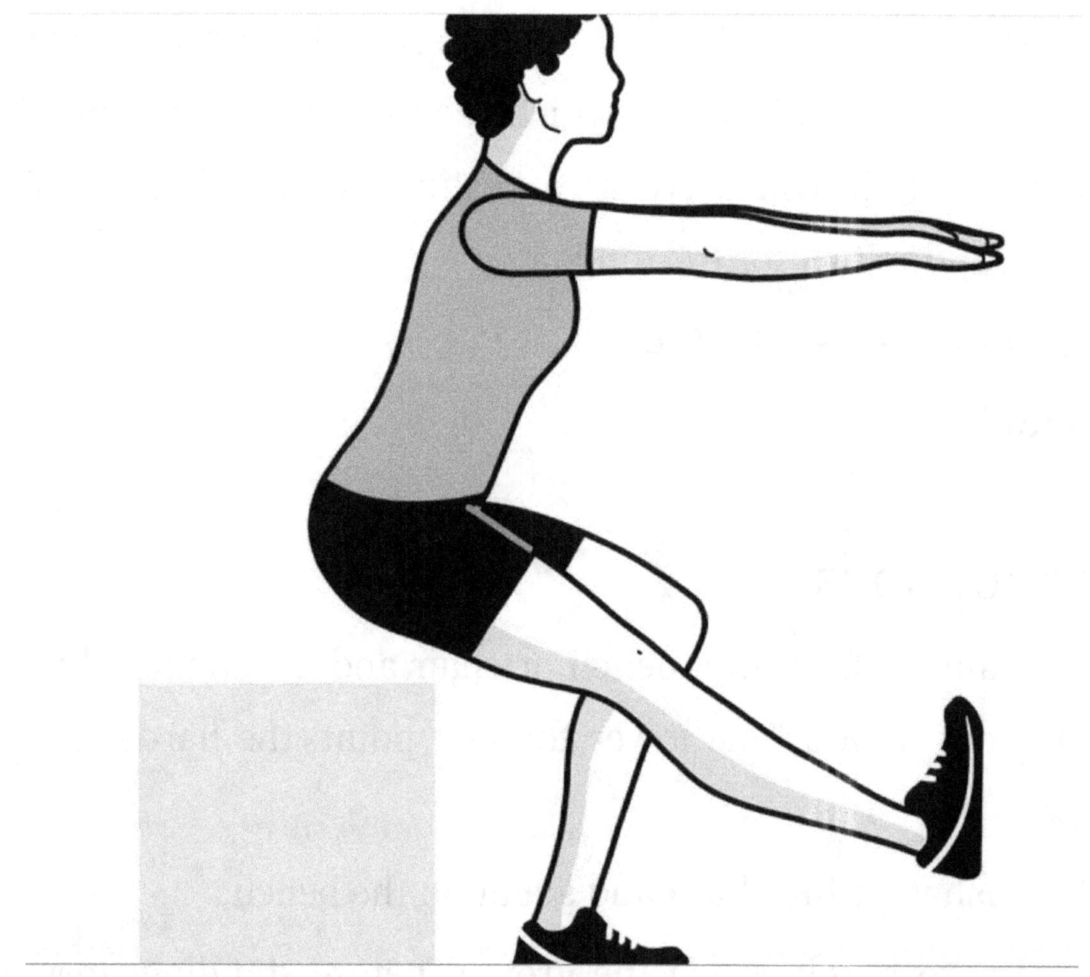

SPLIT SQUAT (WITH BODYWEIGHT OR DUMBBELLS)

The split squat targets the same leg muscles as the squat but places additional tension on the core, knees, and hips, which helps with overall functional strength.

Muscle groups: Buttocks

Quadriceps

INSTRUCTIONS

1. If you are using dumbbells, make sure you are holding them, with your arms dangling by your side.

2. From a standing position, take a long step forward as if you were doing a lunge. The heel of your rear foot should be raised.

3. Keeping your torso upright, slowly lower yourself down until your back knee is almost touching the floor and your front thigh is as parallel as possible.

4. Push back through the heel of your front foot.

5. Complete all reps on one leg and then switch to the other.

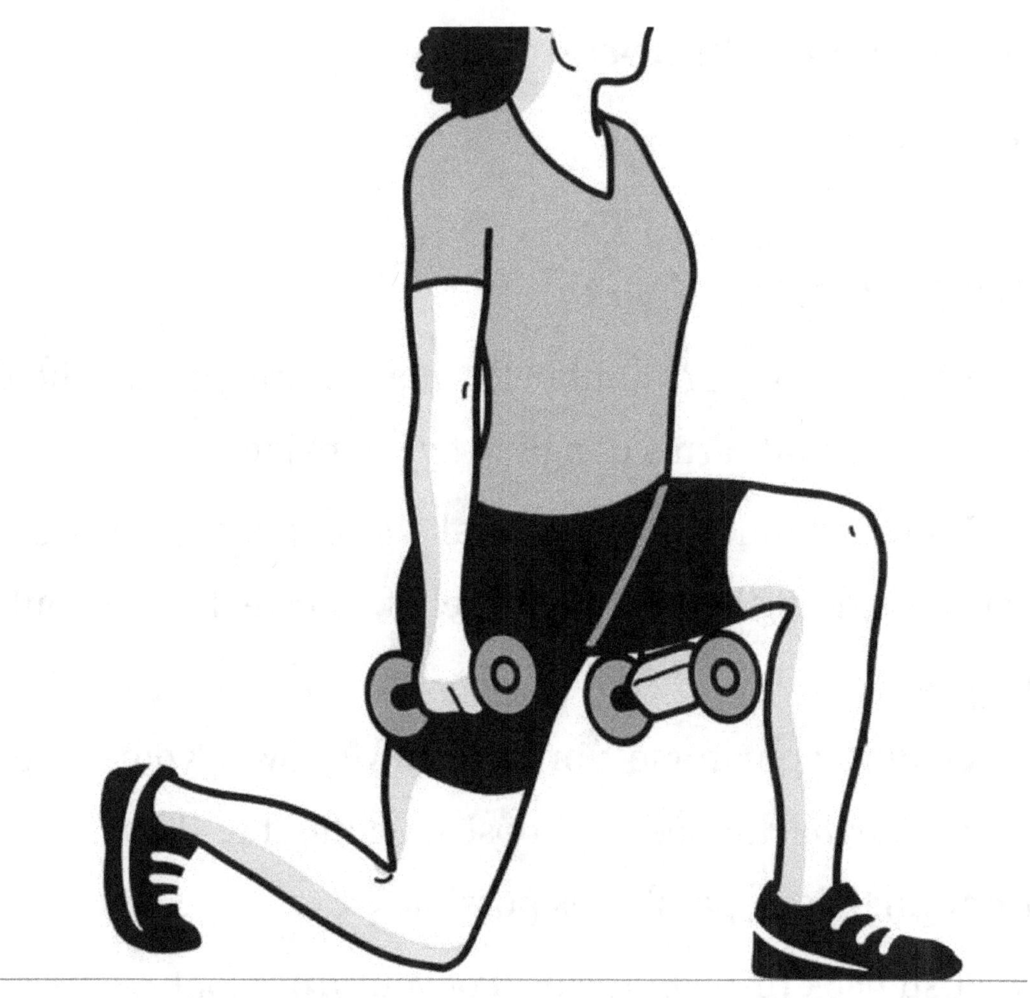

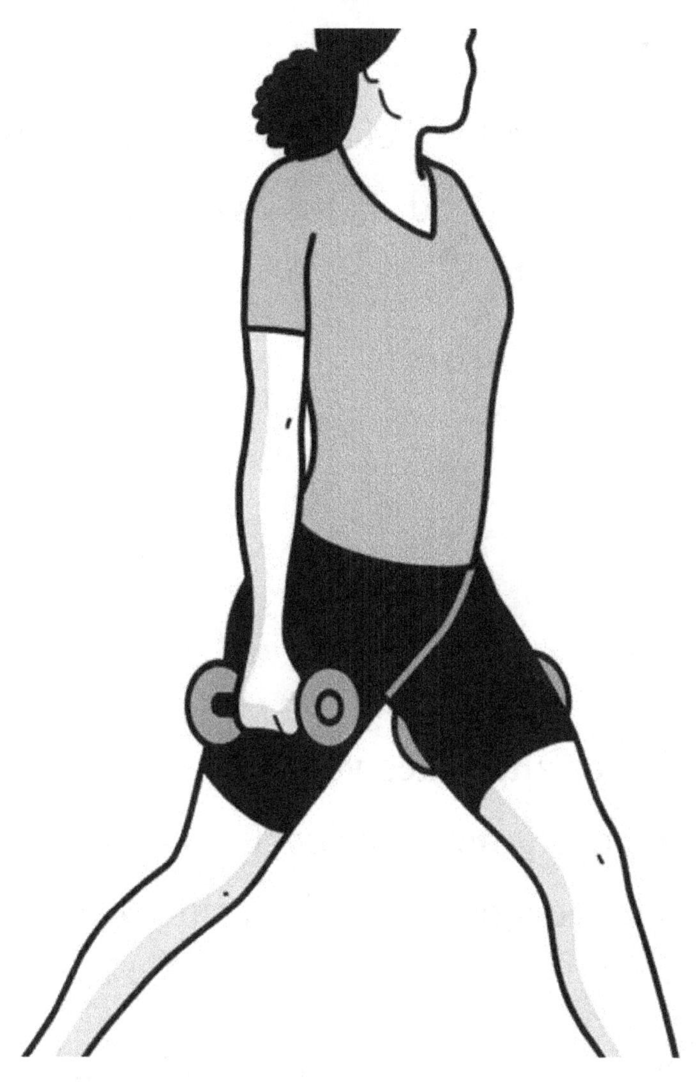

GLUTEAL BRIDGE

The gluteus maximus (often referred to as the glutes) is the largest of your muscles and helps you stand upright and supports your lower back.

Muscle groups: Abdominal

Buttocks

Hamstrings

INSTRUCTIONS

1. Bend your knees and place your feet on the ground, close enough that you can touch your heels with your fingertips as you stretch your arms to your side. Your feet should be hip-width apart.

2. To make the exercise a little more challenging, bend your elbows 90 degrees so that only your upper arms are on the ground and your forearms point towards the ceiling. Otherwise, place your arms on the floor at an angle of about 45 degrees from your body.

3. Drive through your heels and upper back to lift your glutes off the ground. Bring your hips as high as possible,

squeezing your buttocks tightly. Don't push your heels back. Make sure you drive straight up and that your knees don't sag.

4. Squeeze your glutes for a second or two at the top and lower them all the way down to the ground before repeating up to the desired number of reps.

Safety tip: You should feel this movement in your glutes and hamstrings but not in your lower back. Keep your navel pulled so you don't hyperextend your back.

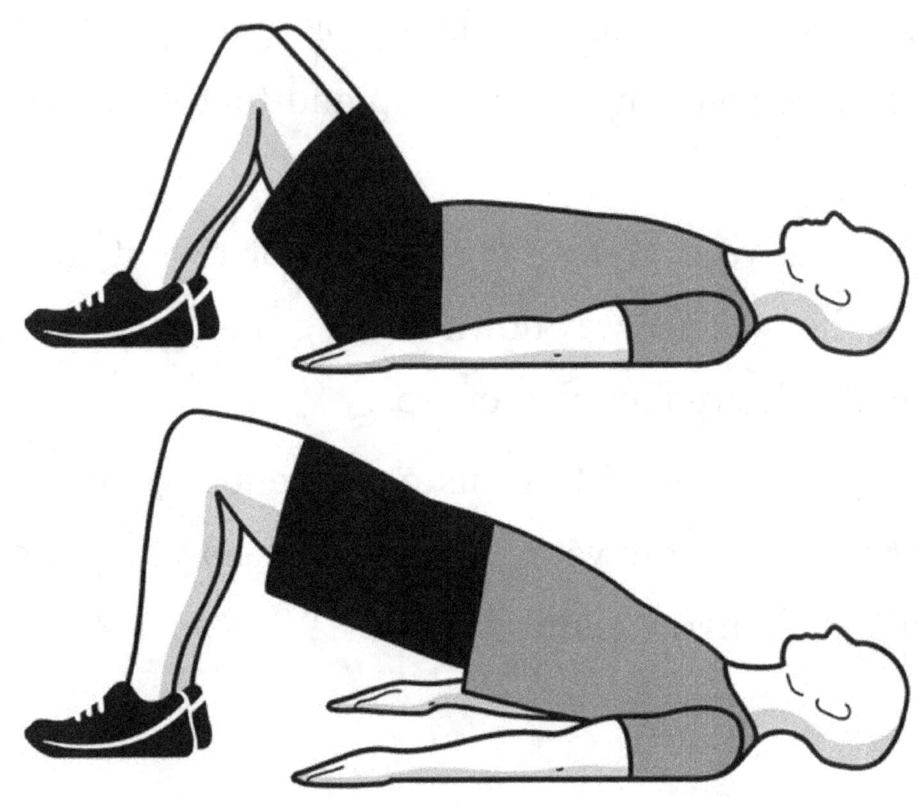

SINGLE BRIDGE IN BUTTOCKS (FLOOR OR BENCH)

This exercise can be performed on the floor or with the upper back on a weight bench at the gym.

Muscle groups: Abdominal

Buttocks

Hamstrings

INSTRUCTIONS

1. Prepare as you would for the glute bridge and then lift one leg off the ground.

2. You can either bend the raised leg 90 degrees or point the toe towards the ceiling. Just make sure you don't swing your raised leg as you lift.

3. Drive through your heels and upper back, lifting your hips as high as possible.

4. Hold up and then lower your back.

Safety tip: Keep your abs engaged to protect your lower back.

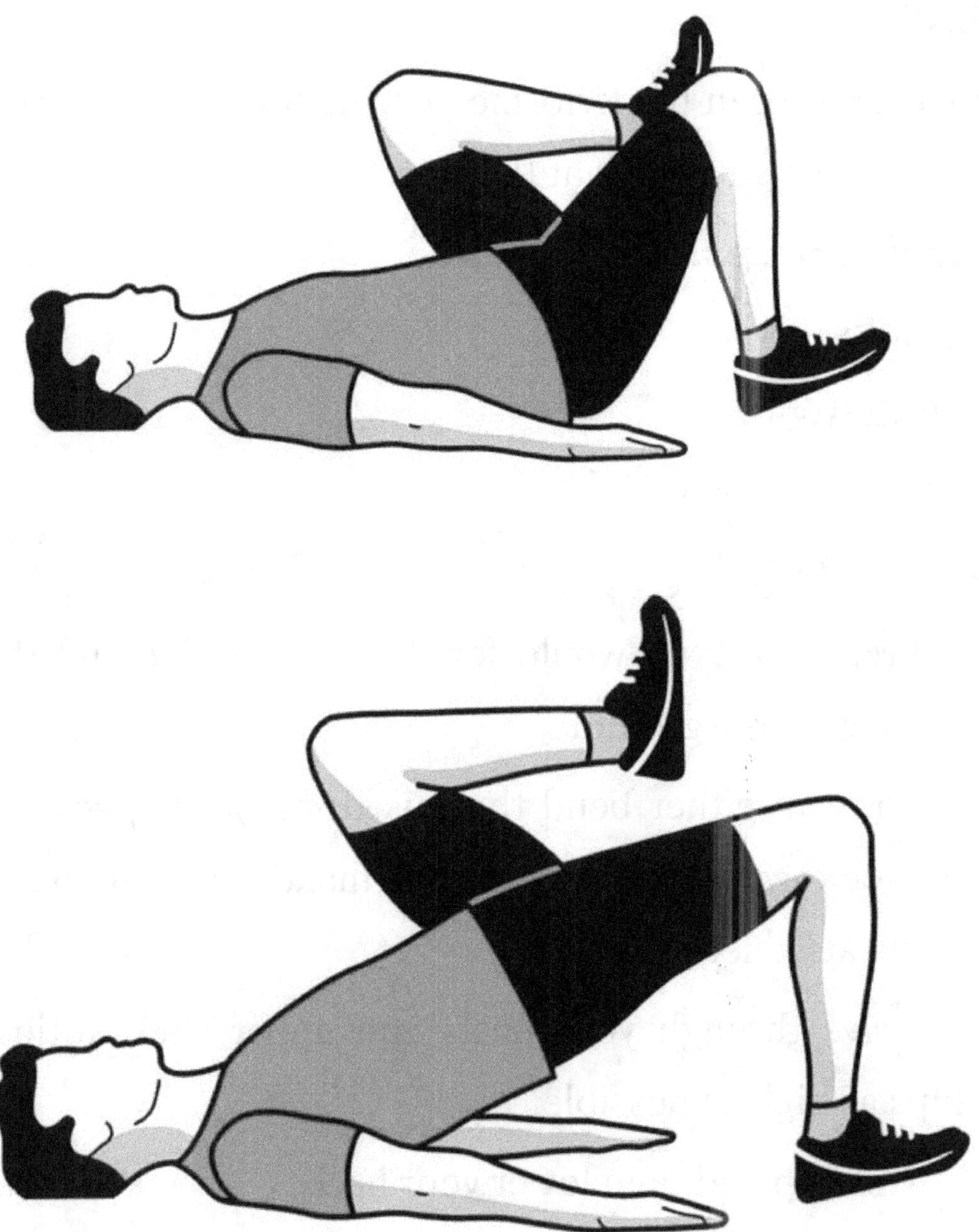

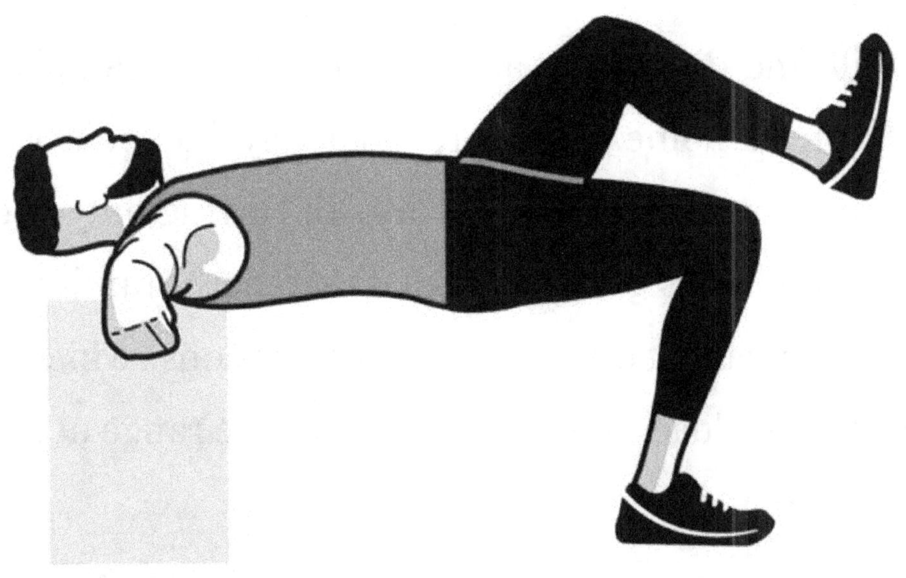

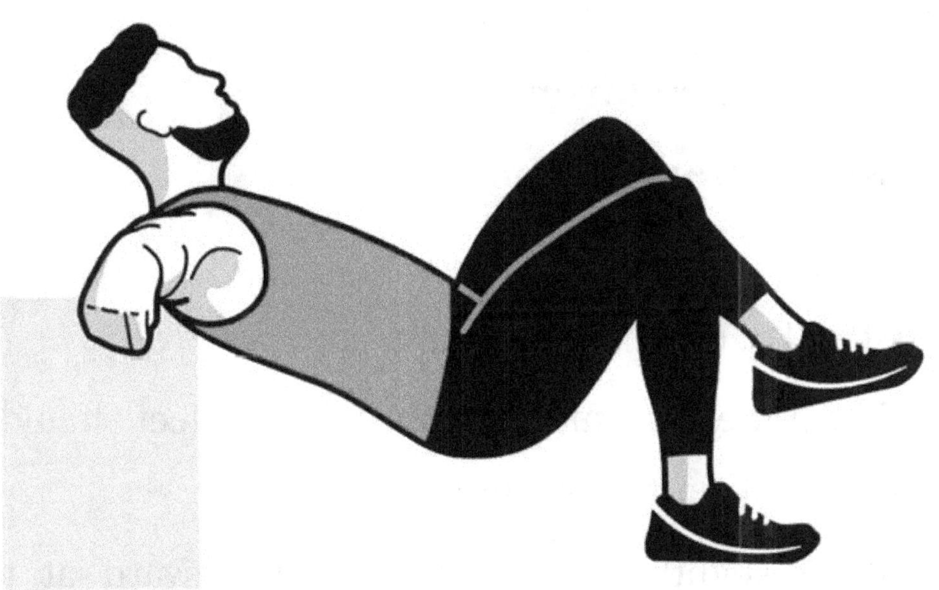

DUMBBELL EXERCISES (FREE WEIGHT)

You will find dumbbells at any gym, but you can also buy and use them at home. They are relatively inexpensive and can easily be stowed under a sofa or bed. Having only two or three sets of dumbbells greatly increases strength training options at home. You can also find adjustable versions, which allow you to change the load quickly, offering a wide range of options.

FOLDED ROW

A classic among strength-rebuilding exercises, the bent rowing machine is a must in your training routine, whether with dumbbells, a barbell or a resistance band.

Muscle groups: Biceps

Latissimus Dorsi Rhomboids

INSTRUCTIONS

1. Begin the movement by placing your feet shoulder-width apart and your toes slightly out.

2. Bend slightly at the knees and forward at the hips. Maintain a reinforced core and a flat back all the time.

3. Driving with your elbows, pull the dumbbells back, bringing your shoulder blades together. Hold this contraction and slowly release to the starting position.

4. Slowly lower the dumbbells. To repeat.

Safety tip: keep your back flat. Do not curve your spine forward.

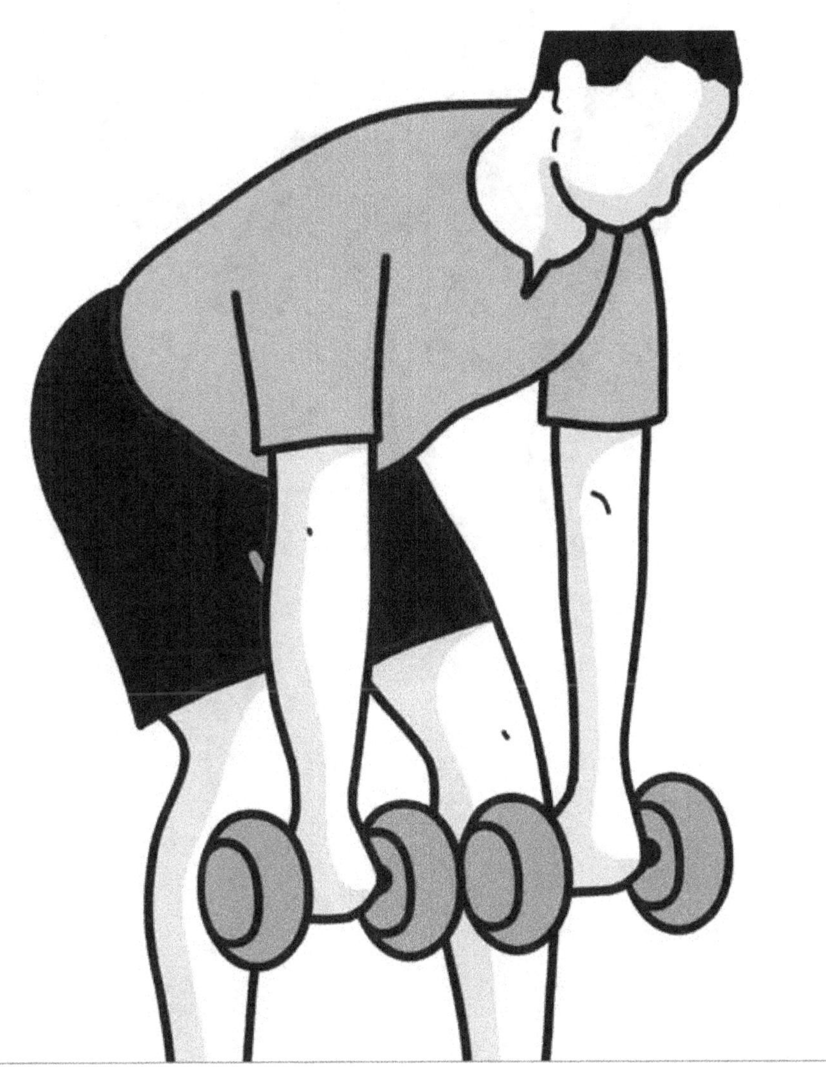

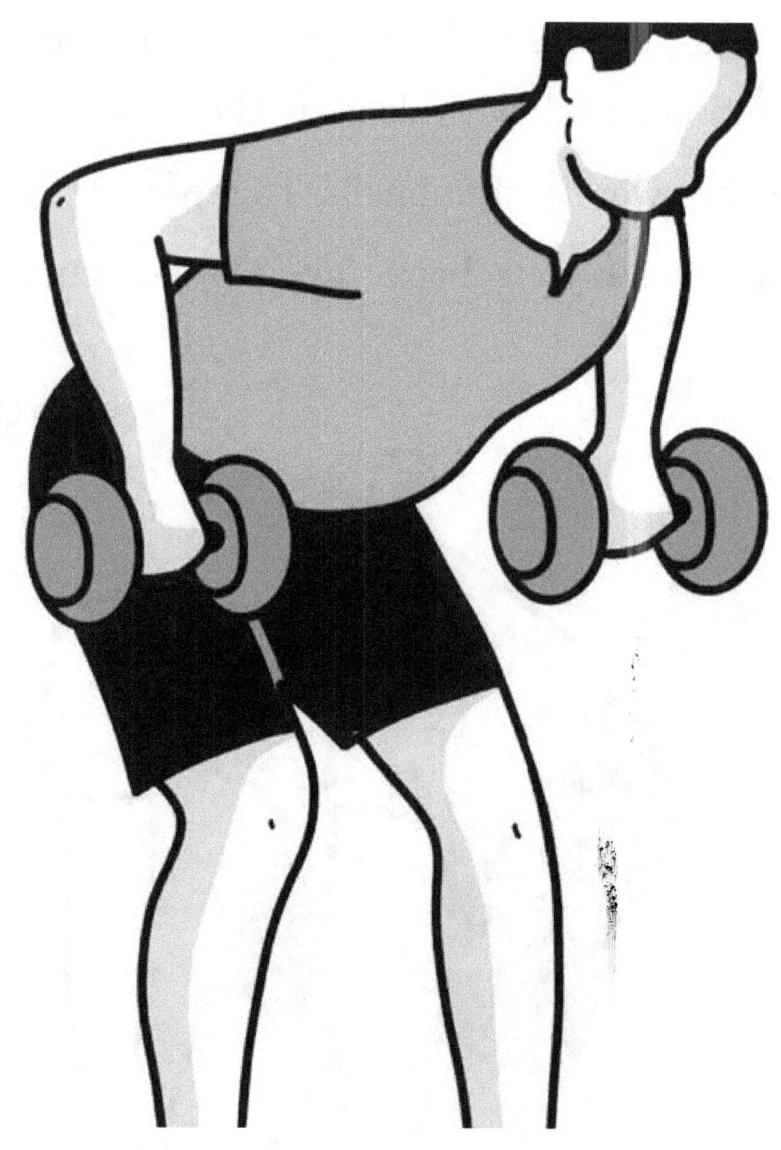

DUMBBELL EXERCISES (FREE WEIGHT)

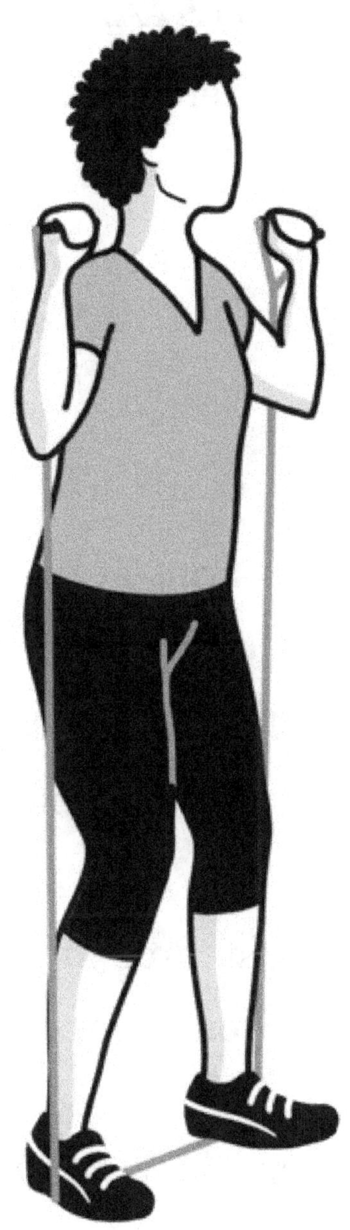

RESISTANCE BAND AND STABILITY BALL EXERCISES

HAMSTRING ROLL-IN WITH STABILITY BALL

This is a simple but effective exercise for strengthening the hamstrings, glutes, and core.

Muscle groups: Abdominal

Hamstrings

INSTRUCTIONS

1. Lie on the floor with your arms at your sides and place your heels on the ball. Press up so that your hips are in the air and your torso forms a straight line.

2. Then, pull the ball towards you, squeezing the hamstrings.

3. Pull the ball back without dropping your hips. It is imperative that you keep your hips raised during the movement.

Tip: You can make it more challenging by placing your hands on your stomach so you can't support yourself with your arms on the floor.

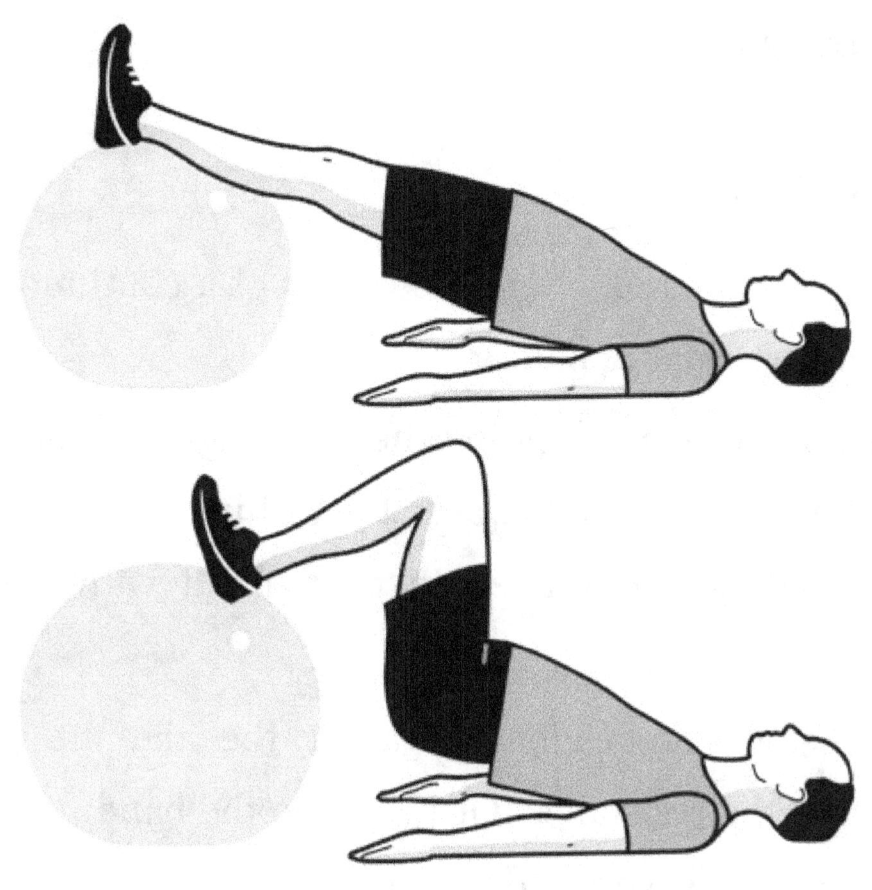

RESISTANCE BAND AND STABILITY BALL EXERCISES

ROMANIAN CART WITH BAND OR DUMBBELL

The Romanian deadlift is an exercise that works on the posterior chain of muscles that run along the back of our body and are responsible for our upright posture.

Muscle groups: Buttocks

Hamstrings

INSTRUCTIONS

1. If using a band, climb the center of a continuous ring or handled resistance band.

2. Bend over while holding the end rings or handles. If you use dumbbells, lean forward at your hips, keeping your back flat, holding a dumbbell in each hand with your palms facing your legs.

3. If using the headband, gather the amount needed to increase the resistance. Or just keep the band further down so that there is very little "play" in the band. (You'll find the point to hold that creates the resistance you need to complete your reps with just the right amount of tension.)

4. With your hips pushed back and forth flat, stand straight while holding the ends of the band or dumbbells.

5. Slowly lower yourself again by pushing your hips back and keeping your back flat until you feel the stretch in the back of your legs (hamstrings).

6. Bend your knees only slightly as you lean forward.

7. Repeat until the desired number of repetitions.

Safety tip: Don't round your back. There is no movement other than the hip hinge. You are not trying to touch the floor.

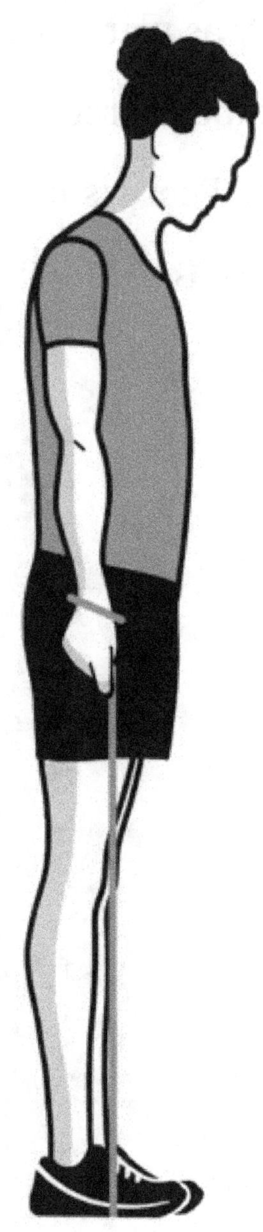

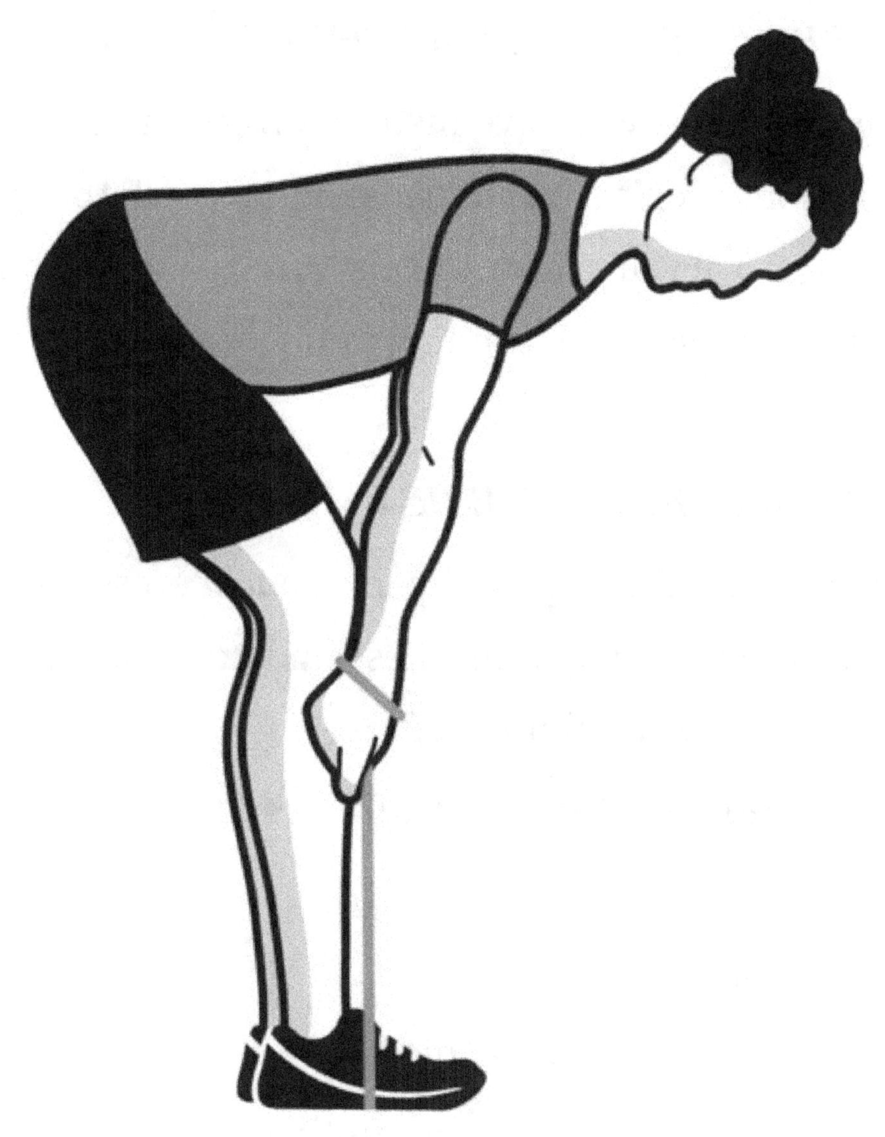

EXERCISES IN THE GYM MACHINE

Most gym machines will have instructions written on them. If the instructions aren't clear, don't hesitate to ask the gym staff for assistance. They are there to help you. Using machines is a safe place to start strength training in the gym.

CHEST PRESS (FIXED RESISTANCE)

This machine mimics a push-up or bench press. It's a safe option for strengthening your chest and triceps, especially if you've never strength training before.

Muscle groups: Pectoralis major triceps

INSTRUCTIONS

1. Sit down and grab the handles.

2. Push the handles forward, until your arms are fully extended but not locked.

3. Slowly return to the starting position, being careful not to let your arms go beyond your shoulder.

4. Repeat until the desired number of repetitions.

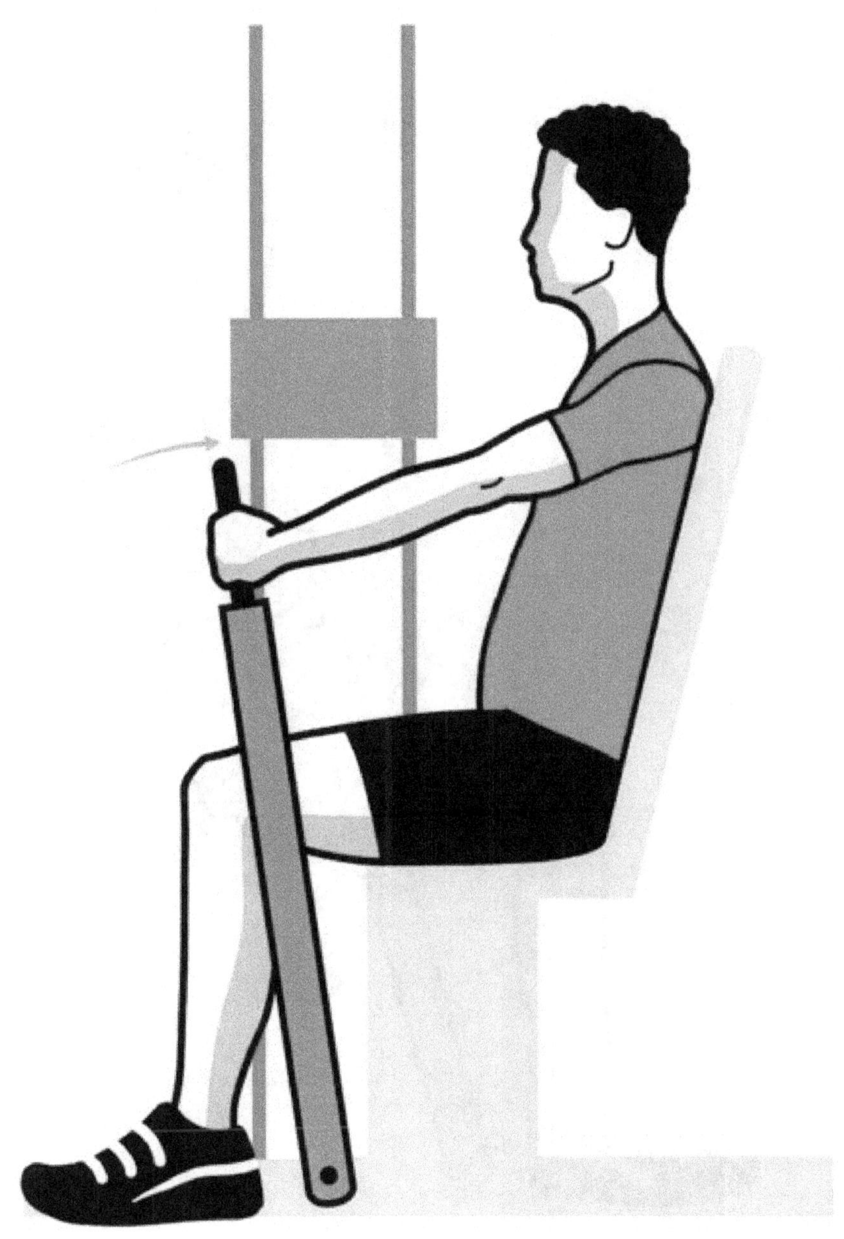

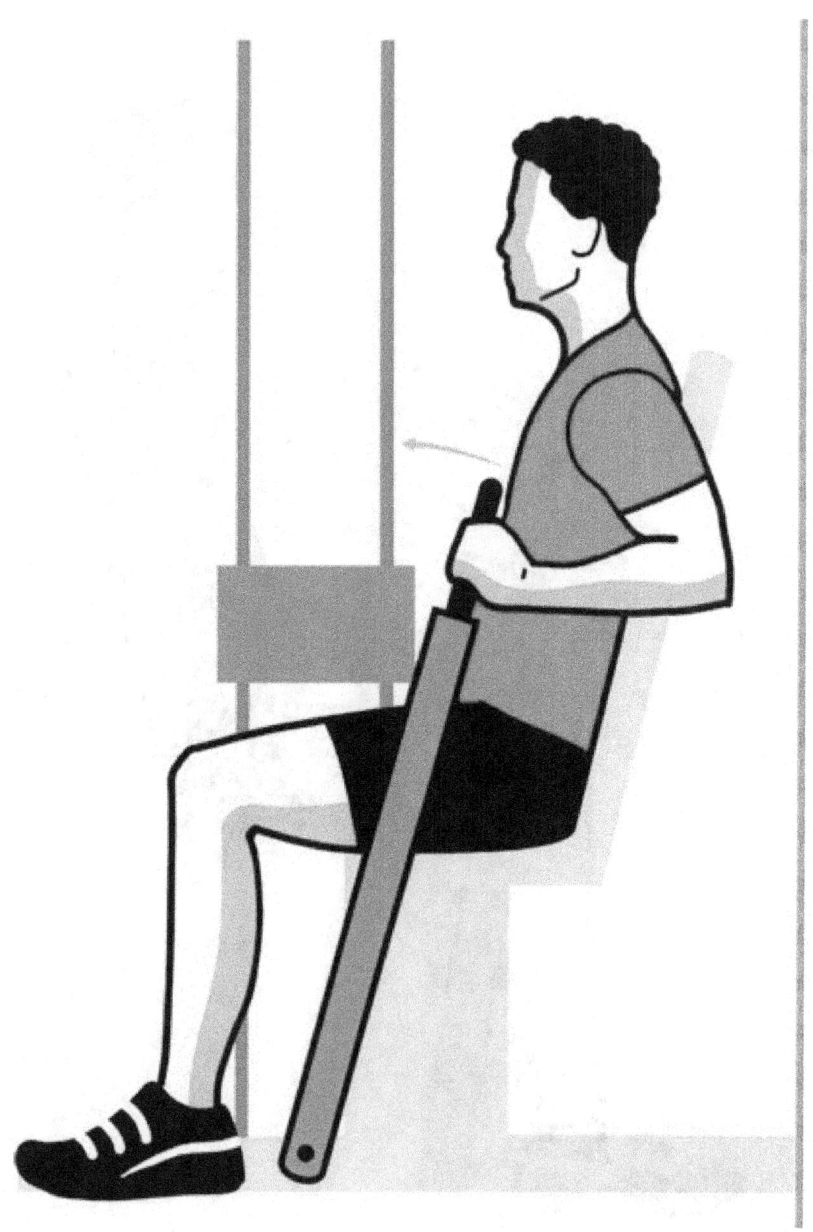

EXERCISES IN THE GYM MACHINE

LAT PULL-DOWN

It's a challenge to replicate this movement at home unless you can do a pull-up, which most people can't.

Muscle groups: Biceps

Latissimus Dorsi

INSTRUCTIONS

1. Adjust the pad to fit snugly against your thighs to minimize momentum.

2. Grab the bar with a wide grip, looking forward with your torso upright. (If you are short like me, you will need to grab the standing bar and sit with it held above your head.)

3. Focus on squeezing your shoulder blades as you pull the bar in front of you towards your upper chest. Resist the urge to lean back to aid movement.

4. Keep your arms at the sides as you pull down, leading with your elbows. Don't allow your arms to move forward as you get tired.

5. Slowly return to the highest position and repeat in slow, controlled movements until you have reached the desired number of repetitions.

6. Tip: Resist the urge to use momentum, swinging back and forth, to help pull the bar down.

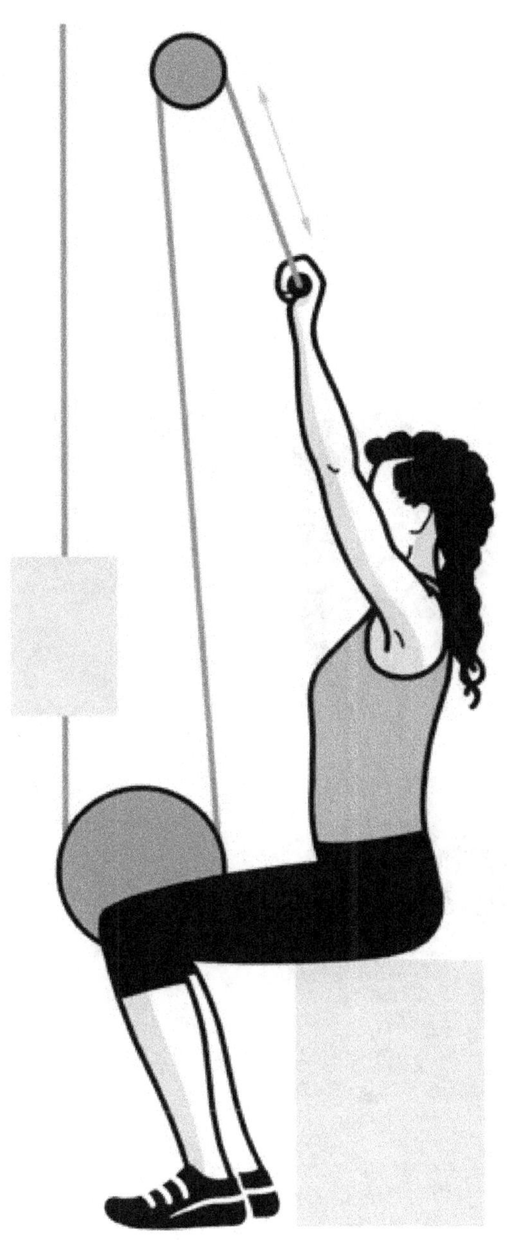

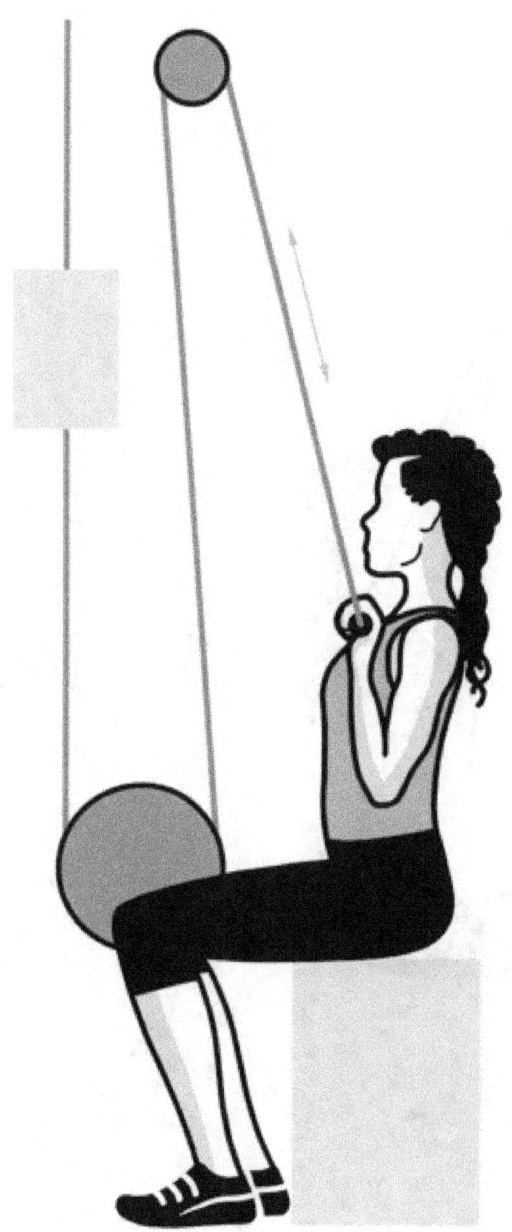

EXERCISES IN THE GYM MACHINE
ROWS OF SITTING CABLES

The seated row of cables develops the muscles of the back and forearms and is a staple among gym goers.

Muscle groups: Latissimus Dorsi

Posterior deltoids

Trapezium

Rhomboids

INSTRUCTIONS

1. Position yourself on the seat with your knees slightly bent so that you can reach the handle with your arms straight. Keep your back flat.

2. Pull the handle and weight towards your lower abdomen while trying not to take advantage of the momentum by moving your torso back and forth. Squeeze your shoulder blades together as you row, keeping your chest high.

3. Bring the handle forward under tension to fully stretch, remembering to keep your back flat even when flexed at your hips.

4. Repeat until the desired number of repetitions.

Safety tip: do not curve your spine forward. Always keep your back flat and avoid using momentum.

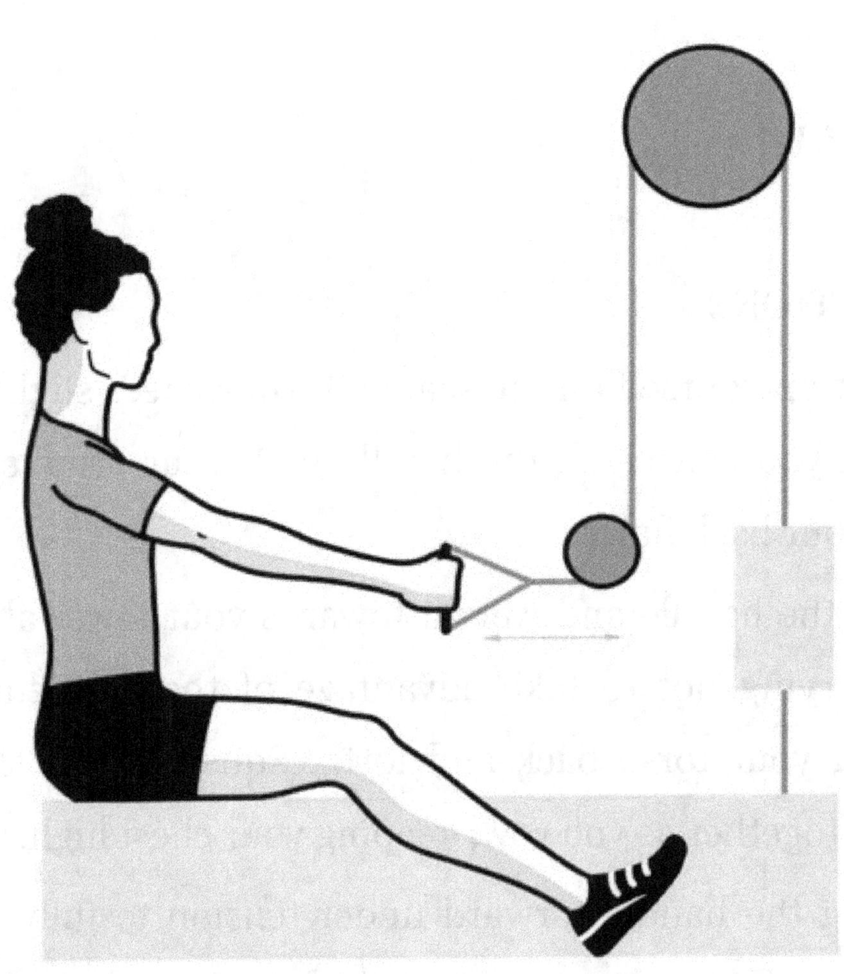

SEAT ROW (FIXED RESISTANCE)

This machine is an alternative to the cable row and dumbbell rows and resistance bands.

Muscle groups: Latissimus Dorsi

Posterior deltoids

Trapezium rhomboids

INSTRUCTIONS

1. Make any necessary changes to the seat or bib. (Most machines usually have height adjustment guidelines and instructions.)

2. Grab the handles by reaching out in front of you. You may have the option of a vertical or horizontal handle. Use whatever feels most comfortable to you.

3. Pull the handles, bending your elbows and pointing them to the sides, while focusing on compressing the shoulder blades.

4. Slowly straighten your arms back to the starting position to complete one rep.

Safety tip: Make sure your wrists do not bend by keeping them in line with your forearm, especially when returning to the starting position.

Chapter 10: SELF TRAINING

One of the things that will ensure you make consistent progress with your workouts is learning the skill of designing your own workout routine and intuitively understanding what works for you and what doesn't. I've mentioned elements of a workout routine in this book so far, but I'll condense it all together here.

The fact is that once you make progress and develop certain levels of strength, chances are you will find that some exercises work better for you, or that some variations make you feel much more comfortable. You may also find that changing the routine itself works better. Wanting to design your own training is perfectly normal.

This is why it is essential to understand how you should do it. There are some elements that go into it. First of all the technical material, it is important to consider the most critical aspect of the exercises and training routines.

Listen

Many people skip training completely or settle for undemanding workouts due to fear of injury. Getting injured and exercising is thought to go hand in hand, and this is an extremely unfortunate development. The desire to continually improve and not get hurt while doing it seems to be at odds with each other, but the reason for this is that there is a serious misunderstanding.

Here's the thing: Your body is constantly communicating with you about how it feels and what it's experiencing. You can choose to listen to it or not. Of course, when you complete mundane tasks like brushing your teeth and so on, you don't need huge levels of input from your body. This is not the case during exercise.

One of the things that makes exercise so powerful is that it not only strengthens you physically, but also develops the connection between mind and body. In other words, you will get to know your body better. More than anything, this is what prevents injuries. Exercise is not an activity like sport. What I mean is that when playing sports, there are many external factors that can cause an injury.

Another player may run into you or you may trip over the ball or any object you are manipulating and, as such, preventing injuries is next to impossible. It usually depends on how lucky you are. In some sports like football or hockey, it is almost impossible to avoid injuries.

Prevention

When you train, you train on your own and have complete control over the movements you choose to perform. The key to training well is to find that zone where you are challenging yourself but not that far from your comfort zone where your body cannot handle the movement.

As a beginner, finding this area is a difficult task. You've probably never exercised for long enough to know the signals your body is sending you. So what are these signals like? As with anything else that has to do with the mind, these signals manifest as feelings. When you try to perform a movement that is well outside your comfort zone, you will feel like it is too hard or uncomfortable.

This is why understanding your body's signals can be tricky. One of the biggest obstacles in the process is distinguishing between the feeling of laziness and an authentic signal. To be honest, they both feel the same for the most part. The difference is in how your body responds to activity and you can think of it as a two step process.

The first step is when you recognize the sensation. The second step is to take action to confirm that feeling. Let's say you are going to the gym and you feel tired or you just don't feel like working out. Your mind is telling you that you better fall asleep or binge on your favorite TV show. Acknowledge the presence of this feeling, but keep doing what you need to do to prepare for your workout.

Once in your training space, which can be at home or at the gym, start your warm-up routine and try out the first set of exercises. This is the crucial part. Notice how you feel at this point. Are you still feeling tired and unable to complete your workout? Has your warm-up left you even more exhausted or fatigued? Or are you excited and find it easy to continue?

The first is a tired case of sincerity, and the second is laziness. Then there is a third confusing case where you will feel tired but still be able to easily perform your workout. In such cases, proceed with caution. It could just be that your body is expending a burst of energy to get you through, or it could be a delayed reaction of your mind before it recognizes that the workout is refreshing. In such situations, it's worth being aware of your movements and not trying to be imaginative with things.

If you're pushing for a new level of performance, take it as slow as possible and make sure you're practicing proper form at all times. Some apprentices sacrifice form to achieve higher levels of strength. If you are an intermediate level trainee (someone who has been training for at least three years), you can do it with confidence as you will know when to curb the habit of breaking form.

As a beginner, you should never break the form, even if it means you can't progress. You should never get pedantic about form, but this is something that takes time to develop. What I mean is that if strength gains are your ultimate goal, sometimes you need to put extra effort into getting past your previous strength levels.

In these cases, you will find that you will not be able to maintain perfect shape. The problem occurs when you get used to it. Intermediate and higher trainees understand that breaking the form for one or two reps is fine, but if they can't perform the movement consistently with the correct form then it's not a real payoff.

Signals

Often you will find yourself in the middle of a workout and your body may be sending a signal that the impending movement is something it cannot do. Again, this is a feeling you will get. You may have completed your pushups easily, but you may suddenly feel that pullups don't seem like a good idea.

It is difficult to tell you exactly what you need to do in such situations because a lot depends on your intuition. In general, here's what you can do. Try the absolute minimum you can for a pullup. This means you hang on to the bar and try to do a half pullup. Don't rush and make sure you are fit. If you still find it difficult to do or if the sensation persists, don't do the exercise.

In such situations, your body has already performed a number of exercises well and this is unlikely to be a case of laziness. So, your body is likely to be communicating that something is wrong with the muscles needed to perform a pull up well. Try the slightest and experience this feeling. Over time, you will get used to the degree of signals and be able to determine if you also need to test the signal.

In general, you should follow a simple principle when it comes to developing your intuition while exercising. To sum it up in one sentence: always do something. This means that, as a beginner, you should pay attention to your feelings and then test them. Since you don't have enough experience yet to understand what they mean, do everything you can and see how it feels.

Never do your training robotic and never treat yourself as such. You are human and your body will progress at the most suitable rate. If Jane next door is progressing faster than you, so be it. You look perfectly fine wherever you are. Fitness is a very personal thing and not something to compare with each other.

You can compare your strength to commonly accepted standards, but that's where it should stop. Don't look at someone who is on a higher level than you and wants to be there. Focus on where you are and everything will be fine. Above all, always listen to your body and develop the mind-body connection.

New movements

Special mentions must be made on the practice of new movements. In these cases, your body and mind are not used to it and, as a result, they don't know what will cause an injury. You will feel discomfort when practicing them, and just as you must learn to distinguish between laziness and intuition, you will have to distinguish between the discomfort that comes from unfamiliarity and intuition.

As a general rule, take it slow when it comes to exploring new movements. Practice the form with as little weight as possible before going all in. Observe your breathing and how your body feels when you perform the movement. As I said earlier, you want to find that area where you are pushing your limits but not that far from where you will injure yourself.

Your intuition will let you know where it is, so trust that you will build it over time. In the meantime, slow down and be aware of the movements you are making.

Your routine

The structure of your basic routine has been outlined above as well as the progression you will follow. Take the time at this point to review it. You will perform the appropriate variation of each exercise outlined in this book so far for appropriate repetitions, starting with (4,4,4) or (3,3,3) if that variation is too hard. To progress to the next level, you will need to perform (8,8,8) or (12,12,12) on certain exercises. Here's what your basic workout routine would look like. Repeat this every other day or whenever you feel rested enough to do the workout properly.

Exercise	Series / repetitions
Dynamic warm-up routine	10 minutes
Appropriate variation for squat progression	3 sets of 4 to 8 repetitions; Rest between one and two minutes between sets
Appropriate pull up variation	3 sets of 4 to 8 repetitions; Rest between one and two minutes between sets
Appropriate variation of the	3 sets of 4 to 8 repetitions;

vertical pushup	Rest between one and two minutes between sets
The appropriate leg increases the variation	3 sets of 4 to 8 repetitions; Rest between one and two minutes between sets
Appropriate pushup variation	3 sets of 4 to 8 repetitions; Rest between one and two minutes between sets
Appropriate Bridge Variation	3 sets of 4 to 8 repetitions; Rest between one and two minutes between sets
Static stretching routine	10 minutes

That said, if you are an intermediate trainee and are already performing at a high level, you can tailor the workout routine to suit your needs. In general, repetition ranges of up to five are suitable for strength training programs. The intervals between five and eight are in the realm of strength / hypertrophy.

Hypertrophy refers to a training process that forces the muscle fibers to become thicker and, as a result, the muscles increase in size. The rep range for strength / hypertrophy ensures that you train for strength and size. Even if you don't maximize either, you will receive the best of both worlds, so to speak.

The repetitions of pure hypertrophy range from 8 to 12. Repetition numbers above 15 are endurance oriented. One thing to note at this point is that as you increase the number of reps you perform, the weight you can lift will also decrease. To build muscle, you need to lift as much weight as possible. Resistance training will not build muscle.

This doesn't mean you shouldn't be training your cardio system. It's just that your training shouldn't be optimized unless you're looking to become a professional marathoner. For everyday purposes, strength / hypertrophy range training is ideal.

Rest periods

The rest periods corresponding to each rep range are different. Strength training routines tend to have longer rest periods, which can last up to five minutes and start from two to three minutes. Strength / hypertrophy training requires rest between two to three minutes between repetitions, although you can rest for shorter periods.

Training for hypertrophy requires rest periods of about one minute. Resistance training reduces the rest period even less with some programs such as high intensity interval training with periods of about 15 seconds or so. As you progress, you may be tempted to increase the size of your rest period to allow you to recover better and perform exercises better.

Understand that rest periods are part of the form and are just as important. If you cannot perform the exercise in the correct form after resting for the required period, then it is not a true rep.

Divisions and isolation

As I mentioned earlier, isolation routines (also called splits) are not suitable for a beginner to practice. For intermediate trainers, however, they provide many benefits. The program outlined in this book can be changed into a split program. The benefit of a split routine is that you can target your muscles individually and you can load them more.

Since you no longer perform compound movements, your body will recover faster. Standard split routines require workouts four or more days per week versus three days per week for strength routines. This frequency simply corresponds to the time it takes for the body to recover.

Designing a split routine with bodyweight training is a little more complicated as it is not completely possible to isolate the muscles as you can with free weights. As a result, you can follow a two- or three-day split. You could do a two-day push / pull split, which will have you do squats, handstand, push-ups and leg raises on the day of the push.

On pull day, you can do pullups, horizontal pulls, and planks, for example. If you wish, you can add additional exercises, such as deadlifts and dips. I will not go into the intricacies of these other exercises as I assume that as an intermediate apprentice, you will have some prior knowledge of the training. Keep in mind that for a division to work well, you will need access to a gym.

A three day split could be on a rotation, pull and core and legs and core. A great option for supercharging your splits is to superset. Supersets involve performing two or more exercises in quick succession that target the same muscle. This depletes the muscle but provides more strength and increases hypertrophy.

How to create a training plan

Let's say right away that creating a personalized training plan is a time-consuming process. It is easy to write a series of exercises on a piece of paper, but it is completely another thing to do. You will find that your body will respond differently to each exercise and rep ranges, as well as volume, so you will need to adapt accordingly to how you respond to them.

Designing a great workout routine for yourself starts with your existing workout log. Remember how I said you need to track your progress with your workouts and note how many reps of each exercise you are doing? Well, this log will form the basis of your custom program.

Review the exercises you enjoy and make a list. Classify them based on push versus pull, as well as the areas of your body they target. Almost every bodyweight exercise is a compound movement, so for the most part, you'll need to make sure there's a balance between the push and pull aspect.

If you find an imbalance between pushing and pulling, you have two choices. You can find alternative movements to compensate for the ones you don't like, or you can suck it and do the ones you don't like.

Next, you need to understand your repetition method.

Reps

There are several methods to implement a repetition range of exercises. You can do supersets, pyramid-style reps, or classic reps. The repetition method used in this book is the classic style of repetition. In this method, the number of repetitions remains constant, as does the weight.

Pyramid-style reps vary in both weight and number of reps. In general, the number of repetitions increased or decreased by two. So you could have (8,6,4) or (4,6,8). As a result the weight is increased or decreased. Cases where the weight has decreased (that is, the repetitions have increased in the sets) are called inverse pyramids. These are considered to be the best when it comes to strength / hypertrophy programs as you will be lifting the heaviest weight when you are cool and the lighter weight as you become more exhausted.

Designing a series of pyramid repetitions with bodyweight exercises is difficult. One option you have is to perform several variations of the exercise for different repetitions. For example, you could do four diamond pushups, six regular pushups, and eight assisted pushups.

Progress

The next element to understand is how you will handle progression and stall. Stall can be controlled by lowering the variation one notch or decreasing the number of repetitions. The progression is a little more difficult to understand. You already have a pattern when it comes to the classic rep range progression in this book.

Pyramids are more difficult to manage. You can choose to add more reps to each set until it reaches a specified number. For example, you can start with (4,6,8) in the pushup progression and increase the number of reps by one each time you train. Once you reach (6,8,10), you can increase the progression level and return to (4,6,8) for this higher level.

In other words, you started out by doing diamond pushups first. You will perform the next highest progression as the second and the next highest progression as the third set. It's a little more complicated and requires more monitoring. The downside is that you can get better strength gains. As with everything else, there is always a compromise.

Keep in mind that your exercise routine needs to be supported by good nutrition principles and the right amount of sleep and water consumption. The more elaborate workout routine will fail if you don't get enough sleep, eat right, or drink too little water.

CONCLUSION

Whether you are a beginner or over 50 or even 70, getting fit is not a complicated process. Sure, it takes work, but that doesn't mean it's impossible or you can't make it happen. It all starts with understanding the basics of exercise and how strength building works. More importantly, you should understand why you need to prioritize.

Next comes an understanding of the three fundamental factors that determine your overall fitness: food, water, and sleep. It sounds so simple, but it is often ignored by most people. Ensuring that you tick the boxes regarding all three will do a lot more for your health than any form of exercise you can undertake.

As you do this, you will need to start exercising. This book has given you a great routine to start with as well as giving you pointers on how to understand where you need to start. Each exercise in this book targets a large group of muscles, so your whole body will receive a full workout.

Remember to perform all exercises with perfect form as this prevents injuries and also increases effective strength. You will be tempted to take shortcuts, but these will not bring about any real change. Your earnings will be temporary and will fade away at the slightest hint of stress.

There are many variations for each exercise, so take the time to get to know them all. Do them slowly at first and don't overestimate your skills. It's better to start slowly and get steady long-term progression than to have to stop and start all the time.

Finally, I would like to remind you to be patient. You may want immediate gains, but it doesn't work that way. You will need to be persistent and consistent in your efforts. Before you know it, you will be there and you will be a different person.

I wish you all the luck in the world. It is an exciting journey you are about to embark on and it is normal to feel a certain level of trepidation and nervousness. You may even feel some form of excitement! Use it to feed yourself further and remember, nothing is impossible!

Finally, if you've found this book helpful in any way,

an Amazon review is always welcome!